The
W A R
Against
Toenail Fungus

New Tools in the Management of
Subungual Onychomycosis

Dwight Thomas, Ph.D.

Monterey Square Press™
Savannah, Georgia, USA

An Important Disclaimer

This book deals with a commonplace fungal infection of the skin and nails which is easy to diagnose but which has been surprising difficult to treat. While the text necessarily deals with current trends in diagnosis and treatment, it is not intended as a guide to self-diagnosis or as an endorsement of any particular therapeutic regimen. Readers suffering from superficial dermatomycoses are strongly advised to consult with experienced physicians. Although considerable efforts have been made to ensure the timeliness and accuracy of the information presented, no guarantee can be given that this book is free from error, nor any liability accepted for errors which have been inadvertently introduced into the text.

To order additional copies of this book—

Please send a check or money order to:

Monterey Square Press
P. O. Box 366
Savannah, Georgia 31402

The price of $18.95 per copy includes postage and will be honored through December 31, 2005. Georgia residents please add the appropriate sales tax. *All sales are final: we will replace copies damaged in the mail, but cannot issue cash refunds.*

About the Author —

Dwight Thomas, Ph.D.,
is a medical writer who is passionately
interested in microbiology and pharmacology. He attended Emory University in
Atlanta, where he studied biology and the
history of science in the shadow of Emory's
imposing University Hospital. During the
Vietnam War he served in the United
States Army, being stationed overseas in
the Rhön Mountains with the 54th Engineer
Battalion. Subsequently he pursued a
doctoral degree at the University of
Pennsylvania in Philadelphia, with financial
support from the Veterans Administration.

Dr. Thomas specializes in translating
sophisticated medical knowledge *into*
plain English, so that it may be understood
by highly literate readers who are as smart
as their doctors but did not have time to go
to medical school. He is a longtime
member of the American Medical Writers
Association, American Mensa, and Phi Beta
Kappa; and he has been the subject of
biographical sketches in *Who's Who in*
America and *Contemporary Authors*.

Contents

Contents Continued

List of Illustrations

The
WAR
Against
Toenail
Fungus

Chapter One

Trichophyton rubrum
The Dirty Red Fungus

Y ou might think that since we were able to put a man on the moon, we would have learned how to cure toenail fungus a long time ago. Really? The fact is that when the Apollo astronauts landed on the moon in 1969— and for several decades thereafter—we had only cumbersome and largely ineffective therapies for this disgustingly earthy problem. And it's not unlikely that some of the feet taking giant steps for mankind on the lunar landscape carried a sneaky *red* stowaway named *Trichophyton rubrum*. This incredibly durable pathogen has not received its due from science writers. Our newspapers and our TV newscasts abound with little horror stories about flesh-eating streptococci, drug-resistant tuberculosis bacilli, botulism, Salmonella poisonings, new mutations in the AIDS virus, and terribly lethal outbreaks of Ebola fever somewhere in Africa. Let's just forget about all these exotic killer microbes and find a way to get rid of *T. rubrum*!! Unless you have an awfully unhealthy or unusual lifestyle, your chances of falling prey to these highly publicized bugs are pretty slim. In contrast, the unsung *T. rubrum* poses an imminent threat to untold millions of Americans. And it is already on your doorstep. Even now it is lurking invisibly in your bathtub or shower stall, in your bed or on your living room sofa, on your carpet or linoleum floor, in your shoes, in your socks, and in your stockings! This germ will never kill you or get you carried away in an ambulance, but it has the potential to cause you all manner of discomfort, inconvenience, expense, and social embarrassment.

What does *T. rubrum* do? Simply put, it causes **athlete's foot**, the perennial curse of locker rooms, and it's also a major player in **jock itch**, that tormenting fungal infection in a young athlete's groin. Yet the cruelest cut comes when those athletic glory days have started to fade into memory. In persons middle-aged and older, whether former athletes or not, *T. rubrum* tends to infect—and ultimately to destroy—the toenails. No other fungal species does this half so well. In the United States more than 90% of all toenail fungus infections are caused by *T. rubrum*.[1] And it's not even a native American germ! Microbiologists speculate that this superbly infectious species arose in Asia or Africa a century or two ago; since then it has been spreading irresistibly throughout North America and Europe, a silent plague of horrendous proportions. To gain some idea of the magnitude of this alien subversion, you need only glance at the well-stocked shelves in your drugstore or supermarket holding over-the-counter antifungal medications. There are dozens and dozens of these products, all claiming to "cure" athlete's foot or jock itch.

Of course, nobody can promise a lasting cure for *T. rubrum* infections. The fungus is everywhere—the most you can do is to reduce those heavy odds favoring constant reinfection. While we can't eliminate this pathogen from the environment, its identification is easy. *T. rubrum* grows readily in the laboratory: after five days of culture, a distinctive reddish tint starts to appear in the petri dish, allowing a positive diagnosis.[2] This bug's colors are always intensely red, as the name implies (*rubrum* means "red" in Latin). For those of us who are old enough to remember the building of the Berlin Wall or to have sweated through the Cuban Missile Crisis of 1962, that particular color scheme cannot fail to evoke the most ominous forebodings.

All fungi of the genus *Trichophyton* are classified as **dermatophytes**, a broader designation which also includes *Epidermophyton floccosum* and several species of *Microsporum*. The combining terms "phyton" and "phyte" derive from the Greek word for plant (*phyton*), and serve to remind us that although fungi may straddle the line between the plant and animal kingdoms, they grow much like plants. Dermatophytes thus take root in our skin or our hair or our nails. While *derma* is Greek for skin, the genus name *Trichophyton* pointedly alludes to hair infections (*trichos* means "hair" in Greek). The species *T. tonsurans* has in fact evolved to invade our hair shafts; it is the most frequent cause of ringworm of the scalp.

The several *Trichophyton* species and the other dermatophytes are basic organisms; they make the amoeba look like an advanced life form. These parasitic fungi are nonmotile; they cannot move about of their own accord, but depend on external sources of locomotion (e.g., human feet) for their transport. Having no lust for sexual unions, they reproduce by vegetative sporulation. The worldwide prevalence of *T. rubrum* is due to the exceptional persistence of its spores, which can lie dormant for months, probably even years, and still give rise to viable colonies when the proper host comes along. Like other fungi, the dermatophytes are saprophytic: that is, they live on dead or decaying organic matter. You might ask, "How can they infect living people if they only thrive on carrion flesh?" The answer to this question does much to explain why athlete's foot will never spread to your lungs or brain, with fatal consequences.

The outermost layer of our skin, called the *stratum corneum*, is actually quite dead. It is composed of layer upon layer of compacted mummified cells which abound with a fibrous protein called **keratin**. A similar state of affairs prevails with our hair and with our fingernails and toenails. The keratin in our skin is soft and elastic. The keratin in our hair is a bit harder; and that in our nails is the hardest and stiffest of all, owing to the extremely tight bonds between the

mummified cells. *T. rubrum* and other dermatophytes thrive on human keratin. They do not
exactly "eat it" as an animal might eat something,
but rather plant themselves in it and secrete enzymes which break it down into its constituent
nutrients; these are then absorbed by the fungal
cells to support their own growth. Fortunately,
only a few areas on the body's surface are susceptible to dermatophyte invasions. You will
never get athlete's foot on your forehead or your
backside because the *stratum corneum* is too thin
at these sites to support fungal implantation.
Moreover, in most places the outer layer of skin
is being constantly and rapidly shed, sloughed off
in tiny invisible flakes owing to external friction
and the internal pressure caused by new cells
growing out of the basal layer. This shedding
also protects against cutaneous fungi. From a
dermatophyte's point of view, our feet offer the
best residential opportunities. The *stratum corneum* is many times thicker here than elsewhere
in the body. In the spaces between the toes—the
"toe webs" as they are called—the keratin-rich
skin is especially soft, and it is not shed so often.
These intradigital areas are fertile soil for dermatophytes; nonetheless, if you went around

barefoot like your Stone Age ancestors, you probably would not be troubled by athlete's foot or toenail fungus. Shoes, socks, and stockings, conventionally perceived as indicators of progress, have actually been the great incubators of **dermatomycoses** (fungal infections of the skin). Occlusive footwear creates and retains both heat and moisture, producing a sticky tropical environment wonderfully conducive to fungal colonization. Athlete's foot begins most often in the web space adjacent to the little toe, because the configuration of most shoes guarantees that the little toe is going to be pressed forcefully against its neighbor. If by chance you have a few *T. rubrum* spores lingering in this web space, the incubational effects will be comparable to those achieved by a hen pressing down hotly on her eggs, save that what is being hatched is athlete's foot instead of chickens.

The symptoms which typically announce *T. rubrum* implantation on the feet should be painfully familiar to most readers of this book. The soft skin at the bottom of the toes becomes less pliable; it may begin to feel somewhat leathery, then it starts to itch. Finally the *stratum corneum* cracks wide open, exposing the sensitive living tissue beneath. That telltale fissure occurs because *T. rubrum* has dissolved the keratin fibers which normally hold the skin together. Pathology workups are rarely deemed necessary in this commonplace situation, but the presence of dermatophytes can be demonstrated by taking a sample of affected skin and gently heating it in 10% potassium hydroxide. The strongly alkaline solution tends to degrade the human tissue while leaving the fungal cell walls intact. When the processed specimen is placed under a microscope, the pathologist will see elongated branching structures called **hyphae** (from the Greek word *hyphe*, "web"). Hyphae represent the standard fungal organization: they are composed of individual nucleated cells arranged one after another, much like links in a chain. With *T. rubrum* large numbers of small, often tear-shaped spores are generally present on both sides of the hyphal strands, much like birds sitting alongside fences or telephone wires.[3] *Oh those terrible spores!!*

The pathologists who first studied dermatophyte infections under the microscope thought that the dense webs of hyphae seen in advanced

T. rubrum

under a Microscope

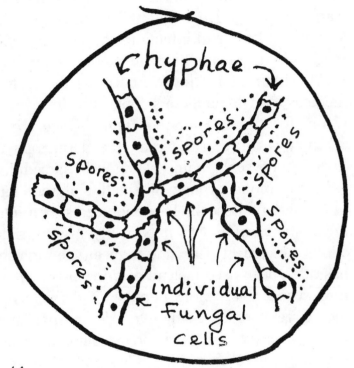

Hyphae are filamentous structures composed of individual nucleated cells.

disease looked like a can of worms. Hence the
generic term *tinea*—that's Latin for "worm"—
came to be applied to all the dermatomycoses.
The particular site of infection was then identified
by adding a second Latinate word. Thus *tinea
pedis* (Latin for "foot") became the proper
medical term for athlete's foot, and *tinea cruris*
(Latin for "thigh") for jock itch. *Tinea capitis*
("head") signifies ringworm, the dermatophytic
invasion of scalp hairs which can spread like
wildfire among groups of small children (e.g.,
kindergarten classes). This book deals with *tinea
unguium* ("nail"), which typically afflicts older
adults. In recent years the term **onychomycosis**
has often been used instead of *tinea unguium* and
now seems to be more popular; it derives from
the Greek—*onyx* being "nail," *mykes* being
"fungus." Both terms are correct, but they are not
perfectly interchangeable. Onychomycosis is a
broader designation which could be applied to
fungal infections of the nails caused by yeasts
like *Candida albicans* or by several species of
mold. These other types of fungi do not have the
same ability to penetrate and destroy the nails that
T. rubrum possesses. While yeasts and molds are
often isolated from mycotic toenails, they usually

prove to be "secondary"—that is, they have colonized the nails only after a primary infection by
T. rubrum or some other keratin-dissolving dermatophyte has already wreaked havoc.

Tinea unguium itself should be viewed as a
secondary infection, since it is almost always
preceded by one or more episodes of *tinea pedis*.
The athlete's foot pathogen initially infects the
unprotected soles and toe webs; only later—often
several decades afterwards—does it set up shop
in the soft keratin-rich underside of the toenails,
presumably gaining entry through tiny cracks in
the nails or in the surrounding skin. Dermatophytes attack previously healthy toenails where
they are most vulnerable, from beneath. Yeasts
and molds are opportunists which settle on top of
previously damaged nails.

American laypersons have increasingly put
their faith in their immune systems to ward off or
to overcome pathogenic microbes. Insofar as
bacteria and viruses are concerned, this attitude
makes a great deal of sense. But it is altogether
wrongheaded with regard to the *tinea* infections.
Because dermatophytes like *T. rubrum* colonize

lifeless structures with no blood supply—the *stratum corneum*, the hair shafts, or the nails— they do not elicit a meaningful immune response. There are no blood vessels to bring protective antibodies or infection-fighting white cells to the sites of these fungal invasions; for all practical purposes, the immune system remains blissfully unaware of the situation. Our hopes must therefore be placed in pharmacology. *Tinea pedis* and *tinea cruris* do not pose a therapeutic dilemma, because just about all the **topical antifungal medications** kept on the open shelves at your supermarket or drugstore can beat back the infection. By "topical" we mean that the therapeutic agent, whether formulated as a cream, a liquid, or a powder, is applied directly to the affected area (from the Greek word *topos*, meaning "place" or "locale"). Killing dermatophytes is easy if you can get your antibiotic to them. The problem with *tinea unguium* is that the fungi are growing in a place which conventional topical agents cannot reach—viz., underneath the nail. There is no evidence that any of the over-the-counter products has significant activity against subungual onychomycosis; they simply cannot penetrate through the nail to the underlying infection.

In contrast, **systemic antifungal drugs** have the potential to cure this condition. These medications, taken orally, quickly find their way into the bloodstream and are subsequently deposited in the keratin of newly-forming nails. The first oral drug used to treat subungual onychomycosis, **griseofulvin**, was greeted with much enthusiasm when it came on the market in the 1950s. But griseofulvin was never very effective against toenail disease: you had to take it every day for over a year, it frequently caused unpleasant side effects, and the cure rates were disappointing.

Because for so many years physicians had no efficacious pharmaceutical therapies for subungual onychomycosis, the malady has given rise to an ongoing parade of **snake-oil remedies**. These products are often hawked in mail order catalogs distributed mainly to older adults. One advertising strategy is to hint that "crumbling and discolored toenails" are caused by poor nutrition (this is almost never the case among well-fed Americans). The topical solution being offered for sale (only ten bucks or so) typically promises to supply "the necessary vitamins and minerals" to "rejuvenate" or to "revitalize" the nails. Moreover, the stuff is "all natural" (but of course!) and "nontoxic" (most certainly). How much do we want to believe this sales pitch! Alas, it is pure baloney for consumption by the gullible, and the product but a placebo.

Another slippery advertising ploy is to convey the impression that a topical antifungal which can cure *tinea pedis* will also work against *tinea unguium*. An advertisement for **Clear Nail®** appearing in a mail order catalog states that this antimicrobial solution "kills all types of nail infections" whether "caused by fungi, bacteria or viruses."[4] We must note that while bacteria and viruses may occasionally infect the nearby skin, they cannot colonize the nails *per se*. If they should ever acquire this ability, we may rest assured that Clear Nail® would take care of them. Of course, the great-grand-daddy of this sales ploy has been **Fungi-Nail®**—an over-the-counter product available in most stores whose very name bespeaks all manner of therapeutic promise. Too much, concluded the Food and Drug Administration in 1994. Subsequently the package insert which accompanies Fungi-Nail® bottles had to cite the FDA's verdict that this topical solution "could not penetrate the nails."

The nonprescription antifungal medications

have the advantage of being relatively inexpensive and readily available. But there are two good reasons why a layperson should not use them to treat apparent nail disease on his or her own initiative. The first is that the disorder may not be due to an infection, fungal or otherwise. **Psoriasis**, a chronic skin disease afflicting several million Americans, often produces abnormalities in the nails which may be hard to distinguish from those caused by *tinea unguium*. Nail discoloration is an early symptom of subungual dermatophyte infection, yet it is hardly a specific indicator. Dermatologists and podiatrists also recognize a **yellow nail syndrome** in older adults. The exact cause remains unknown. While this syndrome is obviously associated with advancing age and a slower rate of nail growth, it has nothing to do with dermatophytes or other microorganisms.

Besides that pressing need for differential diagnosis, another reason to seek professional advice is that recently American physicians have acquired two innovative prescription drugs which hold great promise for the effective management of subungual onychomycosis. **Lamisil® tablets** (Novartis Pharmaceuticals' brand name for oral terbinafine hydrochloride) represents a distinct advance over the old griseofulvin. This drug initially won FDA approval in December 1992; it is the best systemic antifungal we've ever had. Because it is so toxic to dermatophytes, even a short course of therapy (say, three or four months) can stop many cases of toenail fungus. Yet most patients are not going to notice any side effects from Lamisil tablets. **Penlac™ Nail Lacquer** (Aventis Pharma's brand name for 8% ciclopirox solution) is a high-powered topical antifungal which can actually cure subungual onychomycosis in the earliest stage, when the infection is limited to the tip of the nail. Yes, this product does penetrate the nail, at least to some extent. Penlac was developed in Germany and became available in several European countries in the mid-1990s; however, it did not win FDA approval for American distribution until January 2000.

These days most of the M.D.'s and Ph.D.'s who write articles and books about pharmaceuticals seem to have financial and professional ties to the very companies which manufacture and sell these products. Needless to say, when our drug-book author is a large stockholder in the relevant pharmaceutical company or has received considerable *honoraria* (monetary support) from that company, we may suspect that a subtle conflict of interest will inevitably result in an unduly rosy portrait of the product being discussed. As God is my witness, I hereby state that I own no stock in any drug company and have never received a single penny from one. Moreover, I am not engaged in the practice of medicine or in the development and marketing of pharmaceuticals. I must confess that my great admiration for physicians and for innovative drugs is tempered by a healthy degree of suspicion. This attitude is but proper in an independent medical writer who claims no particular credential other than **freedom of the press**—viz., the freedom to write and publish that which is truthful and in the public interest.

And the truth is that neither Lamisil tablets nor Penlac nail lacquer can be honestly described as a miracle drug for *tinea unguium*. Yes, they are much better than previous products, but the course of treatment may still be long and complicated. The regimen which cures one patient may not work with the next; physicians must learn how to tailor the dose and scheduling of these drugs to the individual case of disease. The biggest worm in these shiny pharmacological apples has not been toxic side effects but expense to the consumer. If Lamisil tablets are "magic bullets," they sure are some mighty expensive ammo! You can buy a quart of old Fungi-Nail for the cost of an ounce of Penlac! Yet if you want state-of-the-art weapons in the war against toenail fungus, you must rely on these two new drugs. I know that all too well. For decades I have been fighting off wave after wave of savage *T. rubrum* assaults. And for the past few years I've really been stuck in the trenches—first bogged down in my dermatologist's office—then popping hundreds of Lamisil tablets aimed at the unseen enemy beneath my toenails—and finally hurling bottles of Penlac at that slimy red foe like teeny-weeny hand grenades! *Freedom from this fungus is not free—there's a price to pay.*

Chapter Two

Subungual Onychomycosis
(Learning About It the Hard Way)

What particularly impresses me about contemporary medicine is the tremendous progress we're making in understanding the **mechanisms of disease**. For example, American doctors in the 1970s knew that dread hereditary disorder **cystic fibrosis** simply as a "clinical syndrome"—that is, as a specific combination of symptoms which identified the disease and foreshadowed the eventually fatal outcome. But they really did not know what caused it. These days, of course, we have a seemingly complete knowledge of etiology: we know how a tiny mutation in a gene on chromosome seven causes all the trouble by inducing cells to manufacture an abnormal protein. And we have DNA tests which will tell us whether an unborn child is going to be afflicted with cystic fibrosis. That's a quantum leap in understanding!

Molecular biology also represents our best hope for significant advances in cancer therapy. These days we know how a particular series of genetic mutations will inevitably turn a normal colon cell into a cancer cell which multiplies uncontrollably. Unfortunately, a fuller knowledge of disease mechanisms does not necessarily translate into the immediate introduction of improved pharmaceuticals. Our treatments for cystic fibrosis and metastatic colon cancer still remain largely "supportive" or "symptomatic" rather than truly therapeutic. We have no drug regimens which will cure these diseases.

Anyone who wishes to develop an appreciation for our progress (or lack of it) in the biomedical sciences should browse through the *New England Journal of Medicine* on a regular basis. That's what I've been doing every week for the past fifteen years. Because of this bookish habit, I gradually came to regard myself as the greatest *rara avis* in the world—an informed layperson. Thus you might think that I would have long since learned about the disease mechanisms and presenting symptoms of subungual onychomycosis. To be honest, I was as monumentally ignorant of these topics as the average layperson.

Only much later did I realize that the *New England Journal of Medicine*, like most publications, tends to shy away from the *infra dig* topic of toenail fungus. Shame on the *Journal*! This disease isn't the figment of a hypochondriac's imagination, some vague fatigue syndrome or oh-my-aching-back, but a bona fide microbial infection that you can demonstrate under the microscope. It torments millions; and if we can't anticipate and defeat a dumb adversary like *Trichophyton rubrum*, how are we ever going to cure cystic fibrosis and colon cancer?

Being as clueless as presumably many other *Journal* readers, I reacted with innocent curiosity instead of the appropriate terror when I first noticed a typical presentation of dermatophyte onychomycosis in July 1998. The nail on the second toe of my right foot, next to the big toe, suddenly seemed to have developed a strange bump. There was no pain, nor any swelling or redness in the surrounding tissues, just a little rounded protuberance at the end of the nail. The physicians who specialize in nail diseases call this symptom **distal subungual hyperkeratosis**. "Distal" means at the nail's tip, "subungual" beneath the nail, "hyperkeratosis" an excessive production of keratin. I personally suspect that *hyperkeratolysis* (excessive dissolution of keratin) might be a better word to describe this pathological process. What happens is that the athlete's foot fungus gets underneath the nail tip and secretes keratolytic enzymes which turn the distal nail into a soft spongy mass. The tight bondings of keratin fibers which give the nail its compact shape and its hardness are destroyed, being replaced by a swollen pile of keratotic debris. I learned about these arcane topics empirically when I took a nail file and started to file down that bump on the tip of my second toenail. To my surprise the job only took a few seconds: the elevated portion of the nail quickly crumbled away into a fine powder.

You might ask, "Why is distal subungual hyperkeratosis on the second toe so indicative of *T. rubrum* activity?" To begin with, *tinea unguium* should always be considered as a potential cause of toenail deformity in anyone who has (as I have) a long history of athlete's foot. *Tinea unguium* usually begins underneath the tip of the nail; just one or two nails are initially affected, and these nails are most often found either on the big toe and/or the adjacent second toe. The most frequent location of presentation thus stands in sharp contrast to that of athlete's foot (which usually begins near the little toe), and it speaks volumes about disease mechanisms. Minor traumatic injury to the nail would seem to be a prerequisite for dermatophyte invasion. The big toe and the second toe tend to be affected first because they stick out more than the other toes and are consequently more susceptible to injury. The pertinent trauma probably amounts to no more than stubbing your toe against a piece of furniture, or possibly the constant pressure that your shoe may be placing on that big toenail. And the resulting injury probably amounts to no more than a tiny crack in the toenail or a small cut in the surrounding skin, something which you would not have noticed when it happened and which in any case you could never see without a strong magnifying glass.

Young athletes in their teens, twenties, or thirties often have feet which are hotbeds of *T. rubrum* activity, and they usually subject their toes and toenails to extreme physical stresses. Yet while these youngsters may come down with athlete's foot, they normally are spared the ravages of subungual onychomycosis. The nails in younger persons are strong and resilient, able to withstand most traumatic shocks without damage. And if a youngster's toenail should develop a crack or fissure, the affected portion of the nail usually grows out and gets clipped off before dermatophyte colonization can take place. A slower rate of nail growth is one reason why persons over age forty become increasingly susceptible to onychomycosis. And the toenails are incorrigible slowpokes. In a healthy young adult, the fingernails only take about six months to grow out; but the toenails may need twelve to eighteen months. The growth rate gradually declines with advancing age. In a healthy senior citizen, the toenails can take two years or more to grow out; in seniors with impaired circulation or other chronic health problems, toenail growth may be virtually imperceptible. Should a tiny crack occur in an over-forty toenail, any dermatophyte spores falling into that fissure will have more time to achieve implantation. Alas, older toenails are much less resilient than younger ones, and minor traumatic injury to them is almost a foregone conclusion.

From middle age onward, the nails are less able to retain their moisture content and so tend to become brittle. Persons over age fifty often develop longitudinal ridges (elevated striations) along the entire length of their nails. These ridges do not result from pathology; they are merely a sign of growing older, much like wrinkles on the forehead. And while moisturizing agents and mechanical buffing may improve the appearance of brittle striated nails, these interventions cannot restore that youthful resilience. If older adults chance to harbor a chronic *T. rubrum* infection on the soles of their feet, the odds are excellent that sooner or later they will develop *tinea unguium.*

The medical textbooks cite four different types of fungal nail infections: (1) distal subungual onychomycosis, (2) proximal subungual onychomycosis, (3) white superficial onychomycosis, and (4) *Candida* (yeast) infections.[5] While this conventional categorization must be dutifully repeated here, the author feels impelled to point out that types one and two are really the same thing. Viz., keratolytic disease beneath the nail usually due to *T. rubrum,* the principal distinction being whether the causative dermatophytes first implanted themselves distally (at the nail's tip) or proximally (at the nail's base). Proximal presentations are much less common, but they can occur if the fungi gained access through a cut or abrasion in the cuticle area (i.e., at the "quick" of the nail). **White superficial onychomycosis** is caused by *T. mentagrophytes*, a keratolytic dermatophyte with a different *modus operandi* from *T. rubrum*. This infrequent disease begins on the nail's dorsal surface (its top), the presenting symptom being keratotic debris which looks like a thin coat of white plaster. *Candida* infections often afflict persons with weakened immune systems; they may begin in the moist skin nearby, but then can easily spread to nails that have been damaged by dermatophytes, by exposure to chemicals, by psoriasis, or by trauma.

Types three and four on our list—the superficial *T. mentagrophytes* and *Candida* infections—need not greatly concern us. These diseases are relatively uncommon; an infected person usually notices the problem early on, and it usually can be cured with a topical medication which any dermatologist or podiatrist could prescribe. We are attempting to unravel the Gordian knot posed by subungual onychomycosis. This disease is terribly common, most topical medications have no effect on it, and an infected person may not become aware of it until after irreparable damage to the nail has already occurred. One of *T. rubrum*'s worst attributes is a penchant for insidious advents. The earliest symptom of this dermatophytosis is likely to be a subtle discoloration which can easily be overlooked. The clear pinkish appearance of a healthy nail will gradually be replaced by a cloudy opaqueness or a drab yellow. This change in hue normally begins at the nail's tip and creeps toward the base. But even if you looked at your toenails every day, you would not necessarily notice the alteration with standard room lighting. Those 100-watt bulbs you buy at the supermarket are inadequate; there's a reason why your dermatologist's examining room features a battery of high-powered fluorescent lamps in the ceiling. This specialized lighting does a much better job of revealing that subtle discoloration, yet the most effective illumination for the purpose is Mother Nature's sunshine. Just look at your toenails in broad daylight with a magnifying glass, and you'll have a pretty good idea of whether *T. rubrum* is starting to gain a foothold underneath them.

A lump or any other change in the nail plate which you can feel bespeaks advanced disease rather than a beginning infection. Distal subungual hyperkeratosis, the clinical symptom which caught my attention, requires fungal invasion of the nail plate itself. The nail is subsequently lifted off its bed by the growing mound of keratotic debris. As the disease progresses proximally, the entire nail becomes thickened, soft, and elevated. When it is no longer firmly attached to the underlying tissues, the doctors will speak of **dystrophy** (functional degeneration) or of **onycholysis** (nail destruction). A dystrophic nail is the end product of dermatophyte onychomycosis. The nail now ceases to grow and slowly begins to crumble, starting at the distal and lateral (side) edges. Because the plate is elevated and abnormally loose, it can become painful; and it has the potential to cause infection or inflammation in the adjacent soft tissues. That facile reassurance portraying toenail fungus as a minor cosmetic problem, a song-and-dance offered by all doctors a generation ago and still by some today, is pure hooey. Sufferers from advanced, multiple-nail disease experience discomfort even from well-fitted footwear. Their participation in strenuous pedal activities like running, dancing, or tennis may be hampered. And social embarrassment will keep them from going barefoot to the beach party or jumping into a hot tub with attractive persons of the opposite gender.

At this point the author must inject the obligatory caveat that not all cases of discolored or thickened toenails in older adults are due to dermatophyte activity. Some are simply *idiopathic* (this word gets brought into play when the cause is completely unknown, yet the doctor or medical writer wants to sound knowledgeable anyway). Nonetheless, we should always suspect *tinea unguium* if only one or two nails are initially affected and the rest seem healthy, because *T. rubrum* operates much like the Soviet expansionists of yesteryear. Its march of conquest is surreptitious and sequential: first one toenail, then another, then yet another, all falling mysteriously under its domination like the dominoes once fell in Eastern Europe. (Don't you remember? Estonia, Latvia, Lithuania, Poland, Hungary, Czechoslovakia, Romania, Bulgaria, the list seemed to grow longer every year.) Yes, the **Red Fungus** is much like that; and since its intent is so clear, should we not attack it aggressively at the first symptom of toenail subversion?

My personal opinion is that our scientific data now tend to support prompt intervention with a systemic antifungal drug. The cure of early-stage subungual onychomycosis has become relatively predictable, if not exactly cheap or uncomplicated. It is much more difficult to eliminate the fungal elements from dystrophic toenails; and even if you achieve a mycotic cure, there is little likelihood of ever having normal nails again. Chronic subungual infections can produce permanent scarring in the nail bed and the nail matrix, in much the same way that acne can leave pit marks on the face and tuberculosis can do lasting damage to the lungs. Things are never quite the same.

Chapter Three

The Nail Anatomy Lesson

The average American man rarely gives his nails a moment's thought, unless they get particularly dirty or become painfully diseased. American women go to the opposite extreme. There would seem to be no end to the amount of time and money they are willing to invest in the quest for beautiful nails. Manicures, nail polish, lacquers, polish removers, artificial nails—you name it, the gals will buy it! Of course, the idea that nails are essential for sexual attractiveness has less to do with human biology than with the perpetual advertising blitz conducted by the manufacturers of nail cosmetics. For a moment let's forget about this silly cultural conditioning and consider the real functions that Mother Nature assigned to our nails. In some mammalian species, those hard keratinized structures at the end of the digits are literally a matter of life and death. Lions, tigers, leopards,

and bobcats—the whole genus *Felix* in fact—
need their nails (we call 'em *claws*) to catch and
hold prey; they would surely starve without them.
The same holds true for the American bald eagle
and other birds of prey. With *Homo sapiens* the
fingernails may occasionally be used as weapons
or as grappling hooks, but they are not well
adapted for these purposes. They are instead
little tools which enable us to perform our
constant feats of manual dexterity. Like our
Stone Age ancestors, we still use them to scratch
anything that itches and to remove any insects
(fleas, ticks, lice) which might attach themselves
to our skin. Fingernails do much to explain how
we managed to cover our nakedness, for they
facilitate the manufacture and donning of clothes.
Without fingernails it would be difficult to thread
a needle and to sew, or to tie shoelaces or to
button a button. For those workers whose
occupations place considerable stress on the
fingertips, the nails also serve a protective
purpose. One could hardly be a concert pianist or
a professional typist without sturdy fingernails.

Our toenails are of no use either as weapons
or as tools; their sole function is protection. They
are the helmets, so to speak, which protect the

underlying bones in the toes. When you stub a toe against a piece of furniture, the toenail acts as a buffer which absorbs and dissipates the force of the blow. Without toenails it would be difficult to engage in strenuous foot-oriented athletics like ballet dancing or the broad jump. The odds would be very good that you would either fracture the bones in your toes, or that these bones would damage the surrounding soft tissues. Toenails are important even for such routine functions as walking and wearing shoes. Persons with healthy toenails tend to be oblivious of this fact, but they quickly come to appreciate it when a traumatic injury or fungal infection deprives them of one of these digital helmets.

All medical students face the chore of mastering basic anatomy before they are permitted to think about therapeutics. That's also our situation. Fortunately, nail anatomy is quite simple compared to that of, say, the cerebral cortex (the brain's gray matter). And it is the same both for the multipurpose tools capping our fingers and for the durable helmets capping our toes. The proper anatomical term for the individual nail and all its supporting structures is **nail unit**. We call the hard component that you feel and see the **nail plate**. The plate is created by a group of highly specialized cells called **onychocytes**, in their workshop called the **matrix**. You can't see the matrix: this little pocket of teeming onychocytes is located beneath the **proximal nail fold**, the bit of skin between the nail plate and the distal joint in your finger or toe. The matrix is adequately supplied with blood; and the onychocytes in its deeper portions are very much alive, constantly dividing, manufacturing and stashing away more and more **keratin**. As we already know, it's the well-aged keratin in our skin, hair, and nails which makes them a target for dermatophytes like *Trichophyton rubrum*. The freshly-made keratin in the matrix onychocytes represents our best hope for therapy, because this protein will readily absorb a systemic drug like griseofulvin or ter-binafine (Lamisil) from the bloodstream. The drug is then incorporated in the newly-formed nail plates, where it retains its antifungal activity for several months. Traces of any minerals or metals in the blood are similarly preserved in the nail plate. Those disgruntled husbands or wives who murder their spouses with small intermittent doses of arsenic are not exactly committing the perfect crime. Arsenic leaves telltale transverse lines on the nails, enabling an alert forensic pathologist not only to diagnose poisoning, but to estimate when it began and how often the doses were administered.

In the uppermost regions of the matrix, onychocytes undergo a terminal transformation. They stop dividing and lose their nuclei; at the same time they form extremely tight bonds with each other, almost as if they were glued together. The nail plate now being formed will consist of layer upon layer of anuclear mummified cells, just like the *stratum corneum* of the skin. But a nail can be a hundred times as thick as the *stratum corneum*; and the farther it moves away from the matrix, the harder and thicker it becomes. When we finally see the new nail plate, it is slowly sliding forward over the **nail bed**. This living tissue directly beneath the lifeless plate plays a major role in subungual onychomycosis and thus merits our attention. Being sandwiched between the plate and the underlying bone, the nail bed is of necessity thin. While it receives a constant blood supply, it is not copiously vascularized. The bed's most important function is adhesion—viz., holding the plate in place—yet it also contributes sheets of keratinized cells to the plate's ventral surface, its soft underside. The uppermost cells in the nail bed, those nearest the plate, constitute the so-called "horny" or "cornified" layer. For our purposes it should be stressed that these cornified cells represent fertile soil for dermatophyte implantation, because they are dead and full of soft keratin. Moreover, the bed's horny layer is thickest at the most frequent site of fungal entry, right at the distal end (tip) of the nail plate.[6]

Not all physicians who treat onychomycosis seem fully aware of how intimately the nail matrix and the nail bed are related. Both the matrix and the bed have to be functional to maintain or restore normal nail growth. If a nail plate is lost to traumatic avulsion, a new one will soon replace it if the matrix and bed are healthy. But this is not likely to be the case after long-term *T. rubrum* infection. These dermatophytes put down their first roots (hyphae) in the thin horny layer of the bed, before proceeding to infiltrate the ventral plate. The infection progresses proximally—toward the base of the nail. Eventually the entire bed and the superficial portions of the matrix are

THE NAIL UNIT
Cross-sectional View

Free Edge

Proximal Fold

NAIL PLATE

NAIL BED

MATRIX

BONE

* Hyponychium and distal groove

Living onychocytes in the deeper portion of the matrix create the nail plate and the keratinous nail bed.

affected. When a nail plate finally stops growing, we may presume that scarring has already disrupted both the bed and the matrix. Until this circumstance it stands to be much more difficult to eliminate the infection, and the prospects for obtaining a healthy-looking nail which will grow out normally become exceedingly dim.

The part of the nail plate which we must clip off and which some of us love to bite is called the **free edge**. It is no longer attached to the nail bed, but protrudes into space at the end of the digit. We know exactly where the free edge begins, because it will appear white or whitish yellow in contrast to the "pinkish" plate over the nail bed. In fact, the plate over the bed tends to be colorless and transparent; that pale rosy hue simply reflects the underlying vascularization. Exposure to air brings about subtle chemical reactions in the free edge, changing its coloration to an opaque white. The tough skin which curves downward from the plate at the free edge is called the **hyponychium** (Latin for "beneath the nail"). The tiny crevice between the free edge and the hyponychium is called the **distal groove**. The dirt which accumulates in fingernail distal grooves can be the very devil to remove, as every auto mechanic, gardener, or parent of small active children knows all too well. We don't think much about the toenail distal grooves or worry much about what might be accumulating there. Unfortunately, if you have an active case of athlete's foot, these grooves may be harboring large numbers of dermatophyte spores. Normally the bond between the nail plate and the hyponychium is tight enough to prevent these spores from penetrating the nail unit. But just bang up one of your toes, and the resulting crack in the plate or loosening of the hyponychial bond will open an invasion route for the massed spores of the Red Fungus! Alas, it will probably be many months, perhaps several years, before you notice that something is amiss.

Certain important features of the nail unit are readily visible; we see them every time we glance at our nails, but do not always appreciate their significance. The **cuticle** or "quick" is the thin band of skin between the nail plate and the proximal nail fold. Adhering tightly to the plate, the cuticle functions as a protective seal which prevents bacteria, fungi, and toxic substances from contaminating the underlying matrix. The **lunula** is the whitish quarter-moon-shaped region at the base of the plate (the word means "little moon" in Latin). It represents the most distal and superficial portion of the matrix; the emerging plate here is not as thick or as hard as it will later become. The status of the lunula can give us hints about a nail's overall health and growth rate. In elderly persons the lunula may be very thin or absent altogether, a reflection of decreased activity in the matrix.

Those tough folds of skin you see on both sides of the nail plate create the **lateral grooves**. These folds and grooves channel the plate's outward growth in the proper direction; like the cuticle and the hyponychium, they also serve to seal off the nail unit from pathogens and toxins. This system usually works fine, but is not foolproof. Physicians use the term **paronychia** to describe any inflammation of the lateral folds and grooves, whether caused by a microbial infection or by an irritating substance. Workers who must constantly expose their hands to moisture, chemicals, or potential allergens frequently suffer from

THE NAIL UNIT
Overhead View

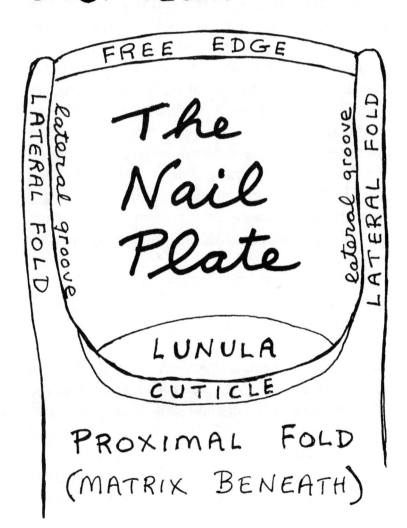

FREE EDGE

LATERAL FOLD

lateral groove

The Nail Plate

lateral groove

LATERAL FOLD

LUNULA

CUTICLE

PROXIMAL FOLD
(MATRIX BENEATH)

fingertip paronychia.   Bartenders, dishwashers, dental hygienists, fish and meat handlers are a few obvious examples. That red rascal *T. rubrum* could conceivably gain access to the nail bed via the lateral grooves, but probably doesn't do so very often. One reason may be that fungal spores are more easily washed out of the lateral grooves than the distal grooves. Another is that the lateral dorsal surface of the nail plate represents a more formidable obstacle to dermatophyte implantation than the distal ventral surface. It's harder and less likely to incur microscopic cracks during a frontal-impact toe stub, the type of trauma which typically predisposes to distal subungual onychomycosis.

The author, who has tried to keep this anatomy lesson brief and painless, will now end it with a word of semantic advice. Your doctor will know exactly what you mean if you speak of the "tip" or "base" of a toenail, but he may be more cordial and forthcoming if you use the anatomical terms ingrained in every medical student's consciousness, yet almost never found in a layperson's vocabulary. Once more for clarity—*distal* means "at a distance from the point of origin" (the nail matrix in this case), and *proximal* means "in proximity to that point."

Chapter Four

My Dermatologist's Office

I am a prisoner of dermatology. For years and years I have been a regular visitor to the office of Doctor P—, a veteran practitioner of that medical specialty. Like other dermatologists, he does not tote a stethoscope in his pocket, but his skill in treating skin diseases is impressive. I had long since come to appreciate his sharp eyes and his thirty years of clinical experience. Doctor P— could accurately diagnose most skin lesions at a glance. And all those unsightly moles and cystic bumps which had been pestering me vanished under his scalpel. Five minutes of painless surgery, and they were gone! "Keep the spot dry for two or three days," he always said, "then clean it with hydrogen peroxide."

Of late Doctor P— has been treating me for certain chronic problems which do not admit of such easy and permanent solutions. First there was the puzzling dermatitis. A strange red rash had suddenly spread across my arms and chest; it did not itch and would not have bothered me much, save that a naive young person of the opposite gender might misinterpret it as syphilis or some other infectious disease. "We don't know what causes that," said Doctor P— with perfect candor as he handed me a prescription for a steroid lotion which could suppress (but not cure) the frequent outbreaks. The actinic keratoses on my forehead and temple represented a more serious matter. In this instance Doctor P— knew all too well what had caused those crusty patches and nonhealing scabs. "Stay out of the sun," he admonished, "otherwise you'll get cancer on your face and back." The several medical dictionaries I keep on my desk turned that Greek diagnosis into plain English. "Actinic" just refers to radiation (from *aktis*, the Greek word for ray). Overexposure to solar radiation tends to irritate the underlying skin cells (the keratinocytes) into an excessive production of keratin; hence those horny areas (keratoses) which are the bane of fair-complected middle-aged sunbathers. A certain percentage of these lesions will ultimately evolve into squamous cell carcinomas, cutaneous malignancies which can destroy sizable swatches of skin and may occasionally metastasize (spread) to other organs. Actinic keratoses therefore need to be treated for cancer prevention as well as for cosmesis (i.e., for appearance's sake). Unfortunately, the first-line therapy calls for the topical application of fluorouracil, a famous cancer drug, to the affected areas. The cream vehicle goes on as easy as Vaseline, but the drug itself is a pharmaceutical blowtorch which quite literally burns off the keratotic skin.

On a dull, dark, and fateful day in January 1999, I found myself in Doctor P—'s waiting room with a face as red as a beet from the effects of that fluorouracil cream. I knew the routine: arrive on time for your appointment, then spend an hour or two up front browsing through deliciously frivolous magazines with titles like *Money* or *People*. Doctor P— treated every dermatological malady in the book, and he was very popular with patients. His front office consequently stayed jampacked with sufferers of every stripe—teenagers with acne or sunburn, adults with herpes or psoriasis, senior citizens with skin cancer. After a decent interval my name would be called, and I would be ushered to an examining room in the rear, where I would pass another half-hour waiting in solitary seclusion. Eventually the door would open, and Doctor P— would enter with a cordial greeting. On this occasion he seemed pleased with the mess—("a good response" he called it)—which the fluorouracil had made of my face. He was just handing me a tube of steroid cream to reduce the inflammation when I mentioned, almost as an afterthought, that something strange had happened to the second toenail on my right foot. "Let's see the problem," Doctor P— suggested. He peered at my naked toes through a magnifying glass. When he looked up again, he suddenly seemed less confident. *"It's the fungus,"* he said ominously.

Doctor P— now left the examining room. He returned carrying a little specimen container in one hand and a stainless steel curette in the other. As I soon learned, the proper technique for specimen collection in distal subungual onychomycosis may require putting the patient through some discomfort. It is usually not sufficient to take a scraping from the top of the nail plate. The specimen should be procured from the plate's ventral surface (its underside) and from the horny layer of the nail bed, because that's where you stand to find the culprit fungi. After the specimen is heated in potassium hydroxide, a quick peek through the microscope normally reveals the telltale hyphae and spores, establishing a diagnosis of dermatophyte infection.[7] The positive identification of *Trichophyton rubrum* as the pathogen requires a five-day culture. This is not often done in routine practice, because it is expensive and would not affect the choice of therapeutic strategies. The same drugs would be used regardless of the dermatophyte species.

Doctor P— did not even wait on the microscopy. He handed me a prescription for **Oxistat**, the brand name of a topical antifungal (oxiconazole) known to be highly active against dermatophytes. "Apply this lotion once a day," he advised, "preferably at bedtime, to that nail and the adjacent big toenail." I asked a damn-fool question in perfect naiveté: "Is this going to clear up the problem?" Doctor P— deftly sidestepped the issue: "Well, it might stop it from spreading." He was now slipping out of the examining room, on his way to the next patient. He paused but a moment to add his customary closing sentence: "I need to see you again in three months."

Chapter Five

Why Me?
The Risk Factors for Toenail Fungus

F inding myself burdened with a diagnosis of appalling gravity, I naturally wanted to learn more about fungal infections of the nails and their optimal treatment. While I admired Doctor P—'s energy and enthusiasm, I doubted that he was the right person to give me the kind of detailed information I sought. For one thing, he was much too busy; by my estimate he saw four or five patients every hour. He was compelled to be efficient, and in various ways he discouraged long conversations. There was also the matter of expense. Being too young for Medicare and not having group health insurance, I had to pay out-of-pocket for my office visits. And those frequent ten-minute consultations were costing me $75 apiece, a rather costly way to learn about disease mechanisms. Doctor P— had impressed upon me the true meaning of the old adage "Time is money." His time—*my money!*

I now turned to the medical libraries and the Internet. Was there really a world-class authority on the subject of toenail fungus, and what did he or she have to say about it? One name seemed to be popping up more often than any other—Robert Baran of the Nail Disease Center in Cannes, France. The French Riviera? I had visions of European royalty and international film stars flocking to that locale on the sly to be cured of this unfashionable malady. Cannes seemed a bit out of my league, both in terms of dollars and of distance. Fortunately, Dr. Baran had just published a book on the topic, written in collaboration with leading dermatologists in England, Germany, and Italy. Several weeks elapsed before my Internet bookseller was able to deliver a copy from the publisher in London. Having plodded through various monumental tomes on cancer medicine, I was relieved that *Onychomycosis* by Robert Baran et al (1999) proved to be a very slim volume (74 pages), the sort of thing you could read in a day or two. Still the book held a few surprises.

Dr. Baran and his colleagues assure us that the odds of developing this disease, like so many others, are strongly influenced by heredity. "*Trichophyton rubrum* onychomycosis frequently occurs in several members of the same family in different generations," observe Baran et al, while pointing out that the disease "is rare in persons marrying into infected families."[8] Thus the mere exposure to *T. rubrum* spores does not inevitably result in athlete's foot and toenail fungus; you also need a certain degree of **genetic susceptibility**. The pattern of inheritance is thought to be **autosomal dominant with incomplete penetration.**[9] In plain English, this means that you can inherit the necessary susceptibility from only one parent, either your father or your mother, and that if you have brothers and sisters, they could be either less susceptible than you are or more susceptible. Dr. Baran and his colleagues postulate that genetically predisposed individuals will tend to acquire a chronic *T. rubrum* infection during early childhood, though the first overt symptoms may not appear until years later.

The longer I studied Dr. Baran's book and other writings on onychomycosis, the more I was able to envision a portrait of the typical sufferer. At length I finally recognized the face which the epidemiologists had painted: it was the same face

I look at in the mirror each morning. Yes, I had all the major risk factors for this disease—I was the perfect candidate. Blissfully unaware of danger, I had always been smack-dab in the cross hairs of the Red Fungus! Did I have a parent who suffered from recurrent *T. rubrum* infections? As far as I know, my mother was never troubled by dermatomycoses; but every morning my father thoroughly dusted his feet and socks with foot powder. After he died of Alzheimer's disease in 1993, I noticed that the electric heater in his bathroom had stopped running. I took it apart with a screwdriver and immediately discovered the reason for the malfunction. The fan and heating coils were covered with a quarter-inch-thick coating of a gummy white powder—and the stuff wasn't cocaine! "Elementary," as Sherlock Holmes might say—foot powder residues in the bathroom unmask the *T. rubrum* sufferer in much the same way that empty booze bottles in the trash betray the alcoholic.

Early childhood? Did I fall prey to athlete's foot at about the same time I came down with chickenpox and the mumps? Oh yes, I vividly remember the tormenting fissure that developed next to my little toe at age eight. A seemingly chronic infection? You bet! During my college days—that's a long time ago—I used a primitive alcohol-based solution to combat the recurring assaults on my toe webs. The liquid burned like fire when it hit those breaks in the skin, and after a few days it stained the skin being treated a bright orange color. Eventually the affected skin would peel off entirely, and I would be free of the problem, at least temporarily. Over-the-counter antifungal remedies have gotten less messy in recent decades, but certainly not cheaper and not necessarily more effective. Nonetheless, you may be sure that whenever I go on a trip, even for a weekend, my suitcase will contain one or more of these nostrums.

Like genetics, the mere fact of growing older was also stacking the cards against me. I had moved well beyond the big Four-Zero, the age boundary at which *T. rubrum* tends to expand its aggression from the intradigital spaces to the toenails. My gender and my occupational history would complete the picture of a patsy. Men are significantly more likely to be afflicted with onychomycosis than women. Their higher incidence rate has nothing to do with the Y chromosome, but with the masculine preference for certain occupations and sports which require occlusive footwear and the utilization of communal showers. The popular name for *tinea pedis* says a lot about the type of individual most obviously at risk—the athletic male who wears running shoes or football cleats for hours on end, then trots off to the locker room for a shower with his teammates. Alas, for someone the least bit prone to pedal dermatomycoses, a communal bathing facility is not apt to be a fountain of purification but a reservoir of disease—the best place in the world to be infected or reinfected with the Dirty Red Fungus. The athlete's foot sufferer who stepped under the shower a few minutes before has washed off more than his sweat and grime: he has inevitably shed microscopic flakes of skin containing viable fungal elements—and these things linger! Dr. Baran and his colleagues provide us with the hardly reassuring data that "*Trichophyton rubrum* survives 25 days in stagnant water at 23 to 25 degrees Celsius."[10] Needless to say, communal showers would be healthier places if they could be constructed so that all the water drained away immediately, and if they were thoroughly disinfected after each individual user. But nobody has invented a practical method for eliminating either the moisture or *T. rubrum* from shower stalls and bathtubs.

If active young men do not become infected in their high school gyms and locker rooms, they have yet another chance when they choose physically demanding professions which require them to wear sturdy shoes or big boots all day long. That heavy-duty footwear is necessary for protection and support, yet has the unfortunate side effect of creating a warm, moist, and snug environment for dermatophyte cultivation. The list of predominantly masculine occupations presumed to be at higher risk due to footwear must include police officers, lumberjacks, telephone linemen, construction workers, mail carriers, and air-conditioning repairmen. It is difficult to find reliable statistics about onychomycosis; but several studies done of coal miners in Germany's Ruhr district in the 1960s and 1970s gave us a striking demonstration of how footwear and communal showers can combine to send the rate of disease incidence soaring upward. About one-third of the miners surveyed had clinically-evident onychomycosis; we're not talking about *tinea pedis* but *tinea unguium*, the final stage of *T. rubrum* infection which is not anywhere so common in the general population. The reasons for the epidemic are easy to imagine: the miners wore heavy-duty boots, they visited the showers to wash off the coal dust before going home, and nobody cared an iota about stagnant shower water or foot hygiene.

Is there any occupation which is even more risky than coal mining? To be sure! Under certain circumstances, military service can be the ultimate risk factor for onychomycosis. A standard American textbook dutifully informs us that "numerous patients associate the onset of disease with military service, especially those stationed for prolonged periods in hot, humid areas wearing heavy, occlusive footwear."[12] Of course, the degree of risk varies not only by the locale of the duty station, but also—and more importantly—by the branch of service. Those dainty white-collar services like the Air Force or the Coast Guard are probably not even as risky as coal mining—why, most service members enjoy a daily opportunity to bathe and to change their socks. Insofar as the risk of *T. rubrum* infection is concerned, Army beats Navy (and the other services) by a country mile. Our occupation of greatest risk is therefore that ultimate weapon—***THE FOOT SOLDIER!***

Let's briefly recount the obvious ways in which the United States Army has offered the best opportunity to contract and incubate a pedal dermatomycosis. To begin with, the Army has always been the largest and most diverse service. Back in the old days of conscription and ridiculously low starting pay, it could never attract enough volunteers to fill its ranks. So it came to depend heavily on persons who were either drafted or who had (like me) "volunteered" a few days ahead of the draft. The Army was of necessity less discriminating than the other services: it accepted all types—the athletic and the sedentary, the aggressive and the meek, the fat and the thin, the Ph.D. candidates and the eighth-grade dropouts, the law-abiding majority as well as certain people whom some judge encouraged to join the Army in lieu of doing prison time. Thus the draftees and volunteers marching into the showers at Army training bases have historically represented the most varied assortment of individuals drawn from all strata of society and from all geographical areas. Needless to say, if there is an especially efficient strain of *T. rubrum* somewhere in the country, we would naturally expect that it too would "join the Army."

'Nuff said about an unparalleled opportunity for pathogen exposure. The opportunity for incubation is also unsurpassed. Combat boots, the standard Army footwear, are the best dermatophyte incubators around. And it's not just that a foot soldier has to wear the same boots day after day, but that frequently he has to wear them for days on end, without an opportunity to wash his feet or change his socks. Even the peacetime Army does frequent training exercises in the field; and the more realistic these are, the less likely that such niceties as foot hygiene will be attended to. Wartime Army duty is fraught with mycotic perils. Being a foot soldier under combat conditions in a warm climate is tantamount to playing Russian roulette with the Red Fungus— and using a six-shot revolver with five chambers loaded! Under this circumstance, the presence or absence of inherited susceptibility to *T. rubrum* doesn't mean much: if you have feet, the odds are excellent that you'll come down with a clinically evident dermatomycosis. During the Second World War, eighty percent of the American soldiers in the South Pacific theater suffered from *tinea pedis* (athlete's foot). Presumably many of these veterans went on to develop *tinea unguium* in later life.[13]

Were there ever any fungi-riskier battlefields than those famous Pacific atolls? Can we point to a more recent conflict which might have some causal relation to the apparent surge in American onychomycosis cases? While Dr. Baran's textbook failed to address these intriguing questions, I found the Internet positively humming with pertinent rumors. "The Vietnam disease," said one website after another. "Vietnam—Vi-et-nam—Vi-et-NAAM!" Naturally I had heard that tune many times before: I had been a foot soldier in the Army during the Vietnam War. Because my experiences in that conflict were so very different from those imagined in the Hollywood blockbusters (*The Green Berets*, *Apocalypse Now*, *Platoon*, *We Were Soldiers*, etc., etc.), I will now relate them as a corrective to celluloid excess. Readers in a hurry for medical information may wish to skip the next chapter; ditto for those who are offended by vulgar language and graphic violence. Others might discover that the boot fits well enough—it is all true, you have my word.

Chapter Six

Memories of Vietnam and Other Wars

D uring the summer of 1969, at about the same time the astronauts were fancy-stepping on the moon, I found myself leaping feet-first into a muddy foxhole set in a comparably craterous yet much more vegetative landscape. It was nearly midnight and pitch-dark; suddenly a break in the clouds allowed sufficient moonlight for me to see a snake rapidly exiting from the far side of the foxhole. *Vietnam?* Not quite but almost! I was a member of Company F of the First Battalion of the First Engineer Training Brigade, based at Fort Leonard Wood, Missouri. Together with two hundred other guys, I was undergoing "Advanced Individual Training" (AIT) as a "Combat Engineer," the Army's particular designation for an infantryman who also knows how to build a pontoon bridge and to set off demolition charges. The ongoing war in Southeast Asia cast a long shadow over our training exercises. "VIETNAM!" screamed the sergeant on the rifle range: "Are you people ready for it? There's only one thing you need to remember—*hit the target or be the target!*" Under the circumstances this advice seemed perfectly reasonable to me, and I blasted away vigorously with my M-14 rifle at the black cardboard silhouettes which kept popping out of the bushes downrange. For all I knew, my life might soon depend upon marksmanship skills. The next silhouettes I might see jumping out of the bushes could be the real thing—onrushing hordes of Vietcong or maybe the NVA, the regulars of the North Vietnamese Army.

As Company F jogged around Fort Leonard Wood that summer, we would frequently chant a little hymn designed to put us in a proper frame of mind. Its verses were easy to remember:

Vietnam—Vi-et-nam—Vi-et-NAAM!

This ditty was not really a song with lyrics, but rather a kind of religious mantra. The constant repetition of the geographical name served as an invocation of Mars, the god of war. I do not wish to convey the impression that the Army entirely neglected cultural acclimation. On one memorable occasion Company F gathered before a thatched hut as a second lieutenant (he seemed barely old enough to shave) explained that the replica was "typical of the construction you see in Vietnam." No doubt he really believed that, but most of us trainees were unimpressed by those portions of our instruction pertaining to the culture of that country or to the rationale for the tremendous American involvement there.   We paid more attention to the course on land mines (just step on one and you'll never need to worry about athlete's foot). And we actually applauded the demonstration firing of a 50-caliber machine gun—it sure kicked up the dust!

After two months of AIT we were as Nam-minded and Nam-prepped as any soldiers could be, and nobody expected the batch of orders we received on graduation day. To be sure, we were being sent overseas—but not to Southeast Asia. Most of us were headed to the Army's private *Sitzkriege*, those less heralded wars of nerves and watchful waiting which had begun long before Vietnam and which would continue long after it. Two nations never mentioned during our training now loomed large on our horizons: South Korea and West Germany. I thought I had drawn the longer straw when somebody told me, "Hey, that APO NY postal address on your orders means you're going to Germany." Europe? I immediately recalled those Army recruiting posters showing a smiling young soldier standing before the Eiffel Tower, with a bright blue sky in the background. Over the next few weeks that image faded away as I began to learn more about my permanent duty station. It was located at a place called Wildflecken, which is not shown on most maps. Nonetheless, if you look at a very large map of Germany, you will discover Wildflecken as a small dot in the extreme northeast corner of Bavaria, right in the middle of the Rhön Mountains. *Wildflecken!* The name means "wild place" in German, but not one German civilian in a thousand will have heard of it. In contrast, virtually all the American soldiers stationed in Germany came to know about it, at least by rumor—or by implicit threat. The word could be applied like a lash to goof-offs and foul-up artists in cushy posts like Aschaffenburg or Hanau: "Screw up one more time, Sergeant Scheisskopf, and you'll go to Wildflecken—is that clear?"

I had no inkling of this forbidding reputation

as I sat in the front seat of a drafty Army truck going down a narrow road which twisted like a snake among steep, densely wooded slopes. Suddenly the forests fell away from the road, and an open vista revealed dozens of massive stone buildings scattered on a hillside. The tall fir trees growing between these buildings almost seemed to touch the dark gray clouds hovering overhead. To the east I could see a formidable mountain with a cross on its summit—the *Kreuzberg*, nearly a thousand meters above sea level and the highest peak in the Bavarian Rhön. The landscape was simultaneously oppressive and wondrous, a scene that might have been imagined in a tale by Edgar Allan Poe, yet it was undeniably real.

Wildflecken—more properly, *die Kaserne* at Wildflecken—was a place built to train soldiers. When I had a chance to walk around the post, I realized that the United States Army had nothing to do with its construction. The barracks were a far cry from the flimsy wooden affairs that the Army had favored for generations, from Fort Laramie onward. These solid two-story buildings had walls that seemed to be about three feet thick, as though someone had wanted to make them relatively bombproof. And those sharply sloping roofs of gray slate still had the little iron hooks which had once secured camouflage nets, so as to prevent aerial observation. In an instant I had solved the riddle of Wildflecken: the entire post was a relic left behind by a previous German Army, not the old Imperial Army commanded by Otto von Bismarck or Kaiser Wilhelm, but the bad *Wehrmacht* which ultimately came to answer to Adolf Hitler alone. The locale's remoteness, its low-lying cloud cover and dense forestation, as well as those telltale camouflage hooks, let me imagine how the United States Army managed to take up residence in a well-preserved Nazi facility. During the Second World War the kaserne had presumably escaped bombing raids because the British and Americans either did not know enough about it, or were not able to observe it very well. On April 6, 1945, American soldiers captured the place intact, lock-stock-and-barrel, after only a minor skirmish with the retreating Germans. And save for the removal of the swastika emblems and the camouflage nets, and a thinning out of the interspersed fir trees, it had remained much as it was.

The burden of a tragic history can be felt in

most places in Germany, and it weighed heavily on Wildflecken kaserne. For me the post came to be both *Denkmal und Mahnung*—a memorial and an admonition. After Hitler reinstated the draft in 1935, the Wehrmacht rapidly expanded its ranks. The military planners wanted a big training area away from the curious eyes of foreign observers, and the Rhön fit the bill. Several tiny mountain communities had to be relocated to obtain the 15,000 acres that the new *Truppenübungsplatz* eventually occupied. Wildflecken was to become the Wehrmacht's third largest facility; those massive barracks were constructed in a single year, 1937, by eight thousand workers who labored round the clock, in three shifts. The Wehrmacht units started to arrive on post in April 1938, often coming in vehicles that were *bespannt* (horse-drawn) as the German Army was not yet fully motorized.[14]

When I arrived at Wildflecken kaserne in September 1969, I had come much too late to enjoy the post's heyday, but right on time for a painful anniversary—exactly thirty years after the German invasion of Poland which marked the beginning of the Second World War in Europe. During the ensuing *Kriegsjahre*, units from all branches of the Wehrmacht (infantry, artillery, armor) trained at Wildflecken, as did certain elements of the *Waffen-SS*, those infamous Nazi warriors whose *esprit de corps* was the embodiment of ruthlessness. We may suspect that the training of soldiers at Wildflecken achieved an intensity far beyond anything that would be permissible on an American Army base. The precise details of this training have not been preserved, though one memorable saying current among the Wehrmacht trainees has come down to us: *Lieber den Arsch voller Zecken als ein Tag in Wildflecken!* "Better a butt full of ticks than a day at Wildflecken!"[15]

You may ask, "Whatever happened to all those young Germans who passed through the kaserne during its swastika era?" Of course, there would probably have been hundreds of thousands of them between April 1938 and April 1945. And we may plausibly assume that most of these new Wehrmacht soldiers received orders sending them to the greatest clash of armies in human history—a land war of almost inconceivable scope and ferocity which made the campaigns of Alexander the Great and Napoleon look like minor squabbles at a tea party. This *Krieg total* began on June 22, 1941, when without warning Nazi Germany hurled a force of three million soldiers and thousands of tanks and planes against the Soviet Union. The American military historian Earl F. Ziemke reminds us that "the fighting lasted for 3 years, 10 months, and 16 days. From autumn 1941 to autumn 1943 the length of the front was never less than 2,400 miles and for a time late in 1942 it reached 3,060 miles." This war was no limited police action like Korea or Vietnam, but an unrestrained fight to the death between the two strongest military powers in continental Europe. A million civilians starved to death in Leningrad after the Nazis blockaded the city. No battles have ever produced higher casualty figures than those fought at Stalingrad and Kursk, each of which proved about five times as bloody as Gettysburg. Dr. Ziemke tallies up the war's human cost in some appalling statistics: over twelve million Russian soldiers died, as did seven million Russian civilians and perhaps three-and-a-half million German soldiers.[16]

The United States, as we know, got off easy in the Second World War. This was not the case with Germany and Russia. The Russian victory in 1945 had the effect of strengthening that country's repressive Communist dictatorship, which was able to stay in power until the 1990s. For Germany this war—like most wars—did not turn out exactly as its planners had hoped. Instead of an expansion of German territory in the East, the opposite happened. *Länder* which had been German for untold generations—East Prussia, Pomerania, Silesia—suddenly ceased to be so. And millions of Germans living in these territories were "encouraged" to migrate westward; they would lose both their homes and their heritage. When the war ended, those massive barracks at Wildflecken kaserne were being used to shelter wounded Wehrmacht veterans. By the end of 1945 the post had been converted into a camp for displaced persons; and the barracks were filling up with thousands of Poles and other East Europeans who had been used as slave labor in the Third Reich, and who were now unwilling to return to homelands overrun by the Red Army. In 1951, as the tensions of the Cold War increased, Wildflecken kaserne once again became an important *Truppenübungsplatz*, this time for the United States Army and its NATO allies.

I knew nothing of the history of Wildflecken kaserne in 1969. I did know that I had been sent to the oldest and most important front line in the Cold War. Why, the border of Communist East Germany was only twenty miles away, an Iron Curtain of barbed wire, mine fields, and concrete watchtowers. And looming behind it was the Red Army of the Soviet Union, which possessed a significant numerical superiority over the NATO forces in West Germany. All roads going east in this region ended in barricades which were topped by warning signs: *"Halt. Grenzgebiet. Nicht eintreten."*

As my days at Wildflecken turned into weeks and months, I began to appreciate the fine irony of my own military career. Instead of sending me to the shooting war in Vietnam, the Army had sent me as far away from that conflict as you could possibly get, unless you joined the astronauts on the moon. It was not just that Wildflecken kaserne happened to be on the opposite side of the globe, but that a blissful silence prevailed. You were not troubled by those constant television images of Air Force planes dropping napalm or of college students shouting in protest. There was no TV at Wildflecken; and with the exception of the Armed Forces Radio, the radio stations were in German. You did not have to read all the hot-airy pronouncements on Vietnam made by politicians and generals, because the English-language newspapers available on post tended to focus on European events.

Duty at Wildflecken kaserne could have other pleasant aspects. The visiting American and NATO outfits who came for a week of training during the summer usually left with fond memories of spectacular natural beauty and sunny days. The career Army people stationed at Wildflecken, the officers and noncoms, also liked the place; they usually lived with their families in quiet residential areas. Unfortunately, Wildflecken kaserne amounted to a tormenting incarceration for the majority of its inhabitants, those low-ranking EMs (enlisted men) who had to live in the old Nazi barracks, sometimes for years on end. These were the "short-timers," the privates and Spec Fours (Specialists Fourth Class) serving in the Army for only two years (if draftees) or three (if volunteers). I knew their plight all too well, for I was one of them. Without a car and with monthly pay of $100 or so, you could not go very far; for practical purposes you were largely confined to base. And your life quickly became a grinding routine of KP, guard duty, and inspections, with an FTX (field training exercise) every other month. That FTX might be conducted in snow or mud, depending on what the weather was doing at the moment. Now you may ask, "Couldn't an off-duty EM catch a bus into town and take in a movie, or maybe meet a girl?" And I will answer: "Are you kidding?" There was no bus and no town to speak of, just a little hamlet of 700 souls down at the foot of the hill. The girls in the vicinity were either Army wives or underage dependents, and therefore off-limits in either case. The post theater did show a new flick once a week; but if you had already seen it, you did not have many other recreational choices. At Wildflecken the principal danger to a soldier's health was not enemy action but the omnipresent combination of boredom and cheap booze. We suffered oh-so-many casualties, almost everybody living in the barracks got hit. The snow began falling in late November and steadily accumulated. Beer bottles tossed into the snow banks outside were promptly covered up and did not emerge again until April, when the spring thaw exposed the evidence of alcoholic carnage and necessitated a cleanup patrol of monumental proportions.

The Army was not devoid of mercy. Soldiers who found their existence at Wildflecken kaserne to be insufferable drudgery were permitted after a decent interval—say, six months or so at this duty station—to file a request for reassignment known as **Form 1049**. In practice, this request would be routinely approved if two conditions were met. First, if the place you wanted to be transferred to was the *Republic of Vietnam*; and second, if you had enough time left on your enlistment to complete a tour of duty in the *Republic of Vietnam*. This reliable escape hatch became a part of our short-timer vocabulary: we would speak of one comrade who had recently "ten-forty-nined" or of another who was in the process of "ten-forty-nine-ing." No further translation needed. We understood that you ran a higher risk of being injured or killed if you volunteered for Vietnam, but this possibility did not trouble us as much as the fatalities occurring in our own neighborhood. German highways were at least two or three times as lethal as American highways. The *Autobahns* had no speed limits and were full of Mercedes-Benzs and Porsches cruising at 120 miles per hour; on those narrow secondary roads you found big diesel *Lastwagens* whose drivers felt impelled to pass any vehicle doing less than 80. A sergeant at Wildflecken had a head-on encounter with one of these onrushing trucks: the twisted mass of metal that was formerly his sports car stayed in our motor pool for many days, an automotive *memento mori*. Teenagers can do awfully dumb things, a proclivity which is not changed by putting them in uniform. One teenage recruit stood up in the back of a flatbed Army truck as it went through a low-clearance underpass; he was nearly decapitated. Another teenager with a visiting infantry outfit pulled the pin on a hand grenade during a training exercise; he neglected to throw it away before it exploded, and there was little the doctors at the post infirmary could do for him.

By January the daylight at Wildflecken lasted only for nine or ten hours, and the snow was three feet deep. I examined a blank copy of Form 1049 at the headquarters of the 54th Engineer Battalion, where my college degree and my typing skills had landed me in a job which kept me out of the snow at least some of the time. I was already stir-crazy, and Vietnam had started to look like an attractive alternative, a kind of daring-do adventure in a sunny warm climate. I now understood why so many Wildflecken EMs wanted to ten-forty-nine: should I join the exodus? I hesitated a moment, then grasped frantically at the hackneyed enticement held out by the Army recruiting posters. While there was a lull in the battalion's FTX schedule, I would take a week's leave and visit Paris. In early February a cab driver from the nearby hamlet ferried me to Fulda, a small city thirty-five miles away, in the German state of Hesse. Unlike Wildflecken, Fulda had connections to the rest of Europe; here you could board a *D-Zug* (fast train) in the evening and be in Paris for the next day's sunrise.

I visited the Eiffel Tower and the other top sights in the French capital, all of which have been lauded *ad nauseam* in movies, novels, and guidebooks, and therefore need not be discussed here. When returning to Wildflecken kaserne, however, I discovered an aspect of European culture which is never mentioned in the tourist brochures yet is not totally insignificant. I had a long layover after midnight, six hours or more, in the Frankfurt *Hauptbahnhof* (main station) as I waited on the first connecting train to Fulda. Having time on my hands, I ventured out to explore the neighborhood, flowing with a restless pedestrian crowd along the broad Kaiserstrasse, then turning left down the Elbestrasse. I had no sense of danger, though the uncanny red glow which emanated from every window and doorway ought to have alerted me that I was entering **A HOT COMBAT ZONE.** Suddenly I found myself under attack—*it was an ambush!* They came at me from all sides, tall blonde girls in black leather pants with open-cleavage blouses. As I later learned, this was the standard uniform of the feared *Strassenstrich Abteilung*, whose spirit of martial aggressiveness has never been equaled by any group of men. I looked for a way to retreat, but I was surrounded. I could only listen to the war cries of ferocious solicitation: *"Schatz! Kommst du her! Ich liebe dich!"* I was almost torn apart, being pulled in opposite directions by two different girls—they were combat-hardened veterans who possessed considerable physical qualifications but not the slightest hint of discretion. At this point I must exercise that neglected quality myself, by imposing a discrete omission upon my text. Suffice it to say, that I went breathless from the scene. Later I realized that Frankfurt's *Strassenstrich* units could recognize American soldiers on sight, even in civilian clothes, and that they would always engage them in mind-to-mind combat. These pitched battles frequently became gland-to-gland.

Back at Wildflecken kaserne those Nazi-era barracks were starting to fill up with returnees from another type of combat zone. The new arrivals had served a tour in Vietnam before they were reassigned to Germany, and in various ways they never let you forget where they had been. They still wore the shoulder patches of their old outfits which had been kicking up the dust in Nam, the "Big Red One" of the First Infantry Division or the yellow horse-head emblem of the Seventh Cavalry. My friend Specialist Wolfe was the worst of the lot. He almost seemed to be polishing his shoulder patch—it displayed the head of an American bald eagle surmounted by the single word *AIRBORNE*. I wondered whether he had ever jumped out of a plane in his life, but yes, he had been attached to the 101st Airborne Division in Nam and so had earned the right to wear that striking emblem of the "Screaming Eagles." I began to feel like a plain Jane in his presence: I wore the blue pentagonal shoulder patch of V Corps, an outfit which had certainly done great things at Omaha Beach on D-Day, but which had not been in a real shootout for over two decades.

A copy of Form 1049 stayed on my desk at battalion headquarters for many months. I never got around to submitting it, and after a while I did not have enough time left on my enlistment for a tour in Vietnam. When I reflect on my service in an Army combat unit during the height of that conflict, I tend to regard myself as a small winner. True, I did not win any medals for valor, but then neither did I get shot or step on a land mine or get doused inadvertently with the Air Force's napalm. Insofar as service-related disabilities are concerned, I long believed that I got home free; of late I have been less certain. Was there a hidden threat to my health lurking somewhere in the poignant shadows of Wildflecken kaserne? Probably—if not the Red Army, then maybe the Red Fungus which can turn your toenails into mush! Microbiologists would certainly concede this possibility. It is not inconceivable that one of those stuck-up Nam returnees picked up a new strain of *Trichophyton rubrum* ripened to virulence in some stagnant rice paddy or fetid Saigon brothel, and then piggy-footed it all the way to West Germany. The shower rooms at Wildflecken could well have been overflowing with the world's nastiest *T. rubrum* spores, courtesy of my friends from the Big Red One and the Screaming Eagles. The paths of glory lead but to the grave—or toenail fungus!

Of course, I know better than to argue a case for onychomycosis disability before the Veterans Administration. The skeptical interrogation that I would be subjected to is not hard to imagine: "You say Mr. Thomas that you were, uh, in the Army during the Vietnam War, uh, but not really in Vietnam, but rather in a Nazi training camp somewhere in the Bavarian mountains, and that you think you were attacked by tall blonde girls and may have been infected with some strange kind of foot fungus?" It's all true, but since when has truth been a pivotal consideration for government bureaucrats? The VA might pay for a psychiatric consultation, but not for the bloody Lamisil® tablets! As a scholar I know that I cannot prove a cause-and-effect relationship between an onychomycotic presentation in July 1998 and Army service twenty-nine years earlier. Ah, but as an author I know that the Vietnam War can serve as a splendid metaphor for *The War Against Toenail Fungus*. This conflict is also going to be inconclusive, inglorious, interminably prolonged, and as expensive as hell.

Chapter Seven

Strictly for the Ladies

B y now I imagine I have gotten myself in hot water with certain distaff readers, on account of perceived gender bias in the last two chapters. I can almost hear the withering critical verdict fired from the feminist lines: "Dumb jocks, coal miners, foot soldiers—of all the silly testosterone-laced foolishness! Don't women get onychomycosis too?" Of course they do—but the ways in which they acquire fungal nail infections can be quite different, so much so that the topic merits a separate chapter. Even the risk factors for toenail onychomycosis caused by *Trichophyton rubrum*, while essentially identical for both sexes, reveal minor variations by gender. Like men, women contract a persistent dermatophyte infection of the feet because they have inherited some degree of genetic susceptibility to the pathogen and have been exposed to it in a communal bathing facility. Fewer women can claim to have been herded through the showers on military bases, yet there are many other perilous locations: swimming pools, poorly disinfected hotel bathrooms, college dormitories, and riskiest of all, the bathroom at home if a family member has athlete's foot, jock itch, or toenail fungus. And while not many women wear combat boots, those high-heeled shoes with the pointed tips may well be equally dangerous. They do a superb job of compressing the toes together, thus facilitating *T. rubrum* incubation in the web spaces. And they may also traumatize the toenails, helping to produce the tiny cracks and fissures which give *T. rubrum* access to the nail bed and the ventral nail plate.

It is not clear which gender suffers the most from fungal nail infections. Men have more cases of toenail onychomycosis; yet women are not only vulnerable to toenail disease but often have fingernail involvement, which is rare among men. The constant battles many women fight to achieve beautiful fingernails are to blame for this disparity. These campaigns can be ill-conceived and mismanaged, more likely to end in a fungal Waterloo than in enhanced sex appeal. Patricia G. Engasser of the Stanford University School of

Medicine points out that nail polish *per se* is not especially hazardous. While some occlusive enamels may retard "the passage of water across the nail plate," these products do form a nitro-cellulose film which is "hard and strong" and protects the plate to some extent. The risk of damage increases when you decide to remove a previous coat of polish. "Chipping off old enamel with another fingernail," Dr. Engasser warns, "damages the nail plate and should be discouraged."[17]   But nail polish removers are hardly better: the solvents they contain tend to extract moisture and lipids from the plate. That weekly routine of taking off the old polish and putting on the new, carried on for decades, may eventually lead to nails which are dry, brittle, and prone to splintering.

Visiting a professional manicurist for nail care is certainly popular—American nail salons gross over six billion dollars yearly—but it can be fraught with microbial hazards. For safety's sake the files, clippers, and other instruments used by the manicurist need to be thoroughly sterilized after each use, just like the equipment in a hospital operating room. Alas, this matter is not regarded with sufficient seriousness either by the manicurists or by the local health inspectors. A survey of nail salons in Houston, Texas, found that pathogenic fungi and bacteria could be cultured from supposedly sterilized instruments in three out of four salons. The researchers doing this survey concluded that the disinfectants used by the salons were relatively ineffective in killing pathogens, and they recommended that "clients should use only their own nail instruments when receiving nail and pedicure services."[18]

Overly aggressive manicuring of fingernails, whether by the individual or by a professional, sets the stage for fungal colonization. Injury or irritation of the cuticle or the nail folds would seem to be a prerequisite for the pathogen most frequently involved in fingernail mycoses, the yeast *Candida albicans*. It is not necessary to visit a nail salon to be infected, as *C. albicans* belongs to the normal vaginal flora. The fact that the long middle finger is frequently involved suggests that the infection may arise after inadvertent or intentional contact with the vaginal reservoir. Fortunately, most *Candida* infections affect the surrounding skin rather than the nail plate, and they can usually be cured with a topical antifungal.

One pathogen which we would not expect to find in fingernail mycoses is *T. rubrum*, whose fief is the feet. Yet women who have substantial toenail disease due to *T. rubrum* often have fingernail involvement as well. The characteristic pattern of infection is known as **the two-feet—one-hand syndrome**, and it speaks volumes about disease mechanisms. The hand affected is the one the patient favors, typically her right hand; presumably she has been using it to pick at the mycotic toenails and so managed to transfer the athlete's foot fungus to her fingernails.

If women kept their fingernails as short as men do, they would be no more troubled by manual onychomycoses than men are. Long nails may be deemed sexy, but insofar as nail hygiene is concerned, they accomplish all manner of bad things. That elongated free edge turns a nail's distal groove into a hard-to-clean sanctuary for fungal spores. It also puts pressure on the entire nail plate and increases the likelihood of trauma to the nail unit. Yet for some people the dictates of fashion outweigh these rational concerns. Women who have difficulty in growing their own overlong nails often turn to artificial plastic nails, which can be cemented on top of the nail plates. A more time-consuming technique is called **nail sculpturing**. Liquid acrylic resins are poured onto the nail plates, allowed to solidify, then molded and filed so as to achieve a fine simulation of elegantly elongated nails. Dr. Engasser observes that these replicas "do not require enamel to look attractive," and that a manicurist can "paint airbrush decorations" on them or "embed jewels" in them. Yet she cautions that the potential risks of nail sculpturing include "irritant and allergic reactions as well as infection."[19] Insofar as the risk of onychomycosis is concerned, any artificial extension of nail length would seem to be even more dangerous than letting one's own nails grow out. *It's just asking for trouble!*

Chapter Eight

Lamisil® Tablets
"The Medicine Stays in the Nail"

By April 1999, three months after my dermatologist Doctor P— had first diagnosed my subungual onychomycosis, I had concluded that the topical medication he prescribed (Oxistat® Lotion) wasn't doing any harm, but then neither did it seem to be doing much good. I was already preparing to tread the well-worn path back to his office when I happened upon a review article in *Archives of Dermatology* which was marvelously apropos to my case. The article, published in the December 1998 issue, had a quizzical title: "How Often Does Oral Treatment of Toenail Onychomycosis Produce a Disease-Free Nail?" Its author Ernst Epstein, a San Francisco dermatologist, assumed the role of devil's advocate when analyzing the clinical trials of the two leading systemic drugs, **itraconazole** and **terbinafine**. Patients are more likely to recognize these products as **Sporanox®** (Janssen Pharmaceutica's brand name for itraconazole capsules) and as **Lamisil®** (Novartis Pharmaceuticals' brand name for terbinafine hydrochloride tablets). Like Dr. Epstein, I could see that the clinical trials done on toenail fungus therapies left a lot to be desired: they were small, enrolling a few dozen or several hundred subjects instead of thousands, and the physicians conducting them tended to use imprecise criteria (e.g., "improved appearance") to measure a treatment's success or failure. Dr. Epstein would have none of this halfhearted fuzziness; his criterion for treatment success was a presumable cure, defined as "a clinically normal nail" shown to be fungus-free by "negative results of potassium hydroxide microscopy and culture." Of the 26 clinical trials he identified, only seven used this combination of "morphological results and mycological findings" as their end point. Analyzing the data from these seven trials, Dr. Epstein concluded that "standard courses of terbinafine achieved a disease-free nail in approximately 35% to 50% of patients." He pegged the cure rate for itraconazole regimens at "about 25% to 40%."[20]

Dr. Epstein's piece cut deep to the dilemmas inherent in our therapeutic strategies. You have to rid the nail plate, the nail bed, and the nail matrix of all viable fungal elements before you can claim a cure; and nobody can be sure just when that cure has occurred or how long it might last. An experienced dermatologist's impression of an improved or clearing nail certainly carries some weight, but then such visual judgments are subjective, and they do not demonstrate the absence of fungi. While a positive culture gives us conclusive evidence of dermatophyte activity, a negative culture doesn't prove the opposite, because attempts to culture these fungi may fail for one reason or another. Microscopic examinations are easier to do, yet fall short of providing certainty. If you see hyphae and spores under the microscope after a course of Lamisil or Sporanox, it is not always clear whether these fungal elements are still alive (treatment failure), or dead and simply waiting to be shed (treatment success). And assuming you are able to cure the first case of subungual onychomycosis, how do you prevent the seemingly inevitable reinfection if the patient is prone to athlete's foot and has the less resilient toenails of middle age?

I cannot say that these problematical issues greatly concerned me as I marched into Doctor P—'s office; instead I felt the smug satisfaction of someone who thinks he has made an important discovery. "I need some Lamisil," I told the cute young nurse who was ushering me into an examining room. She appeared to be impressed by my decisiveness and pharmacological knowledge; I savored her reaction like a glass of vintage wine. About an hour later Doctor P— finally got around to seeing me. His reaction to my proposal, while guarded, was not altogether devoid of enthusiasm: "Lamisil?   Yes, that's the treatment of choice—gets two out of three cases—you have nothing to lose by trying it." Then he seemed to hedge his bets: "Of course I have no objection if you want to continue the more conservative therapy you've been using." I stayed my course— Lamisil it was! Doctor P— handed me a prescription for thirty 250-milligram tablets, with two refills permissible. The standard onychomycosis regimens recommended by the manufacturer call for one tablet a day for six weeks to treat fingernail disease, and for twelve weeks to treat toenail disease.[21] I was going on the twelve-week regimen.   Doctor P— explained that he limited an initial Lamisil prescription to thirty tablets, just to be sure the patient could tolerate the drug before buying too much of it.

I wasted no time in presenting that prescription at a nearby pharmacy which promised fast service and reasonable prices. Well, their service is usually expeditious, but on this occasion I had to undergo a preliminary interrogation before I received the pills. "Mr. Thomas? Mr. Thomas?" I heard the pharmacist calling from behind the counter. "Have you ever taken this medicine?" he asked. I assured him that I knew what the drug was used for, yet I could sense that he was not really interested in testing pharmacological awareness. A second question haltingly un-masked his true concern: "Do you know, uh, how much it costs?" Oh yes, I could pay for it too! The bill came to $242.20—or exactly $8.07 for each modest-sized tablet. When I got home, I did something I had never done with any previous prescription. I counted each pill one by one—and then I counted them again!

Fortunately, apart from sticker shock, there were no other unpleasant surprises awaiting me as a new Lamisil patient. At the low dose levels used to treat superficial fungal infections, this

drug tends to be remarkably free from side effects, and I did not notice any. Doctor P— had
instructed me to take the tablets with food, but
you can also take them on an empty stomach.
Roderick J. Hay, an English authority on Lamisil,
assures us that "the agent may be administered
with or without food or after recent use of antac-
ids." The body's absorption of the drug remains
the same.[22] And whether taken with or without
food, it causes few gastrointestinal symptoms, no
more than 5% of patients being affected. Perhaps
2% to 3% of patients will develop a rash or some
other skin reaction as a result of Lamisil therapy.
In general, when these most common side effects
do occur, they usually are mild and temporary;
and they do not require discontinuation of the
drug.[23]

It is unfortunate that systemic therapy for
onychomycosis has never fully emerged from the
dark shadow cast by griseofulvin, the old antifungal drug which did not work very well and often
caused headaches and nausea.[24] Some physicians
who prescribe Lamisil seem unduly worried
about the potential for hepatotoxicity, those dele-
terious effects on the liver which can occasionally
be life threatening. Lamisil (oral terbinafine) is,

of course, processed by the liver before it reaches the toenails. Dr. Hay observes that "terbinafine is extensively metabolised in the liver, resulting in 15 different, clinically inactive metabolites." About 40% of the ingested drug becomes available as a therapeutic agent "following first-pass hepatic metabolism." Terbinafine is eventually removed from the bloodstream by the kidneys, about 70% or 80% being passed with the urine, the rest leaving the body with the stool.[25]

A healthy liver and fully functioning kidneys are the main prerequisites for uncomplicated and worry-free Lamisil therapy. The drug is a little straw (so to speak) that gets placed on the liver, no problem at all for most people, but potentially back-breaking for a liver whose function has already been compromised by chronic hepatitis or alcohol-related sclerosis. Prospective patients should inform their physician if they think they have pre-existing liver disease, or if they consume large doses of alcohol, acetaminophen, or other drugs which can put stress on that organ. Under these circumstances Lamisil may be counterindicated, and the wise physician will order a blood test to verify hepatic function before considering therapy.[26] Once in a blue moon, somebody has an apparent idiopathic reaction in which exposure to oral terbinafine seems to have precipitated liver failure; the incidence is probably no more than one patient out of several million.[27] For the overwhelming majority of patients taking this drug, the liver function tests are going to come back perfectly normal. Several clinical trials done in the 1990s gave us an idea of what to expect: 3.3% of the Lamisil patients had hepatic irregularities, typically "asymptomatic enzyme elevations." This compares favorably to the 1.4% rate of hepatic irregularities recorded for subjects taking a placebo.[28]

Besides having a high safety profile, Lamisil has a strong claim to being the most effective agent for subungual onychomycosis caused by *Trichophyton rubrum* or by other dermatophytes. In this context it must be compared with Sporanox® (oral itraconazole), which received FDA approval for American distribution in September 1992. Like Lamisil, Sporanox is an expensive drug which has been extensively advertised to the general public as well as to physicians. Both drugs are much more keratophilic than the old griseofulvin. They are readily absorbed by the keratin of the newly-forming nail plate and nail bed, and they retain their antifungal activity in the plate and bed for several months after therapy has ended. This residual action explains why we have been able to develop short regimens for them, three months or so, while griseofulvin therapy typically required a year or more. Both Lamisil and Sporanox are directed against the same general target in fungal cells: they disrupt the biochemical process by which these cells manufacture ergosterol, a necessary component of fungal membranes. But there are important differences between the two drugs. Sporanox belongs to a class of antifungal agents called **azoles**: these interrupt ergosterol synthesis at a late stage and are primarily *fungistatic* in their action—viz., they stop the growth of fungal cells. Lamisil is a **synthetic allylamine**: it specifically binds to and inhibits an enzyme called squalene epoxidase, which is needed at the beginning of ergosterol synthesis. Since Lamisil acts early on, it is not merely fungistatic but potently *fungicidal*: it can kill dermatophytes outright, even when present in minute concentrations. And it has the great desideratum for an antibiotic: it is terribly toxic to the pertinent microbes without noticeably affecting the human host in most cases. Dr. Hay assures us that "terbinafine is highly selective for the fungal squalene epoxidase, with virtually no inhibitory effect on the mammalian enzyme." The prescribing information published by Novartis Pharmaceuticals cites laboratory tests which have indicated that a 4,000-fold higher concentration of terbinafine would be needed to suppress mammalian squalene epoxidase "than is needed for inhibition of the dermatophyte enzyme."[29] Thus when taken in the low doses typically prescribed, this drug is unlikely to reduce the synthesis of cholesterol and other vital steroids in humans.

The laboratory data pointing to Lamisil (terbinafine) as the superior agent against dermatophytes have been borne out by clinical trials. The German trial conducted at the University of Münster and twenty-two other medical centers gave us some representative statistics which are worth repeating. This trial randomized 170 patients with toenail onychomycosis to receive either twelve weeks of oral terbinafine (250 mg daily) or twelve weeks of oral itraconazole (200 mg daily). The cultures done before randomization established that *T. rubrum* was the pathogen in 161 patients (94.7%). *T. mentagrophytes* was isolated from eight patients (4.7%), and *T. violaceum* from a single patient (0.6%). The trial's end point was "mycological cure"—viz., fungi-free nails as documented by "negative results on microscopy and culture." By one year after the start of therapy, 81% of the terbinafine patients had achieved that end point, compared to only 63% of the patients assigned to itraconazole. The German investigators observed that while terbinafine therapy had no demonstrable effect on cholesterol levels, most patients taking itraconazole revealed decreased serum cholesterol "in the range of that which is seen with lipid-lowering drugs." This finding suggests "that the inhibition of sterol synthesis by itraconazole is not completely fungus specific."[30]

Although Sporanox is probably a heavier straw to be placed on the liver, this drug also enjoys a favorable safety profile at low doses and is usually well-tolerated. Yet Lamisil would seem to have a slight edge in safety and tolerability as it does in dermatophyte killing power. Sporanox must be taken with food to ensure proper absorption and to avoid gastrointestinal upset; and since it disturbs hepatic metabolism more than Lamisil, it has a greater potential for unwanted interactions with other drugs that patients may be taking. The manufacturer's prescribing information contains a long list of agents—anticoagulants, antihistamines, calcium channel blockers, cholesterol-lowering drugs, steroids—whose activity may be either increased or decreased by the concomitant administration of Sporanox.[31] Lamisil interacts with only a few prescription drugs (e.g., cimetidine, cyclosporine, rifampin). However, coffee drinkers should be warned that concomitant Lamisil will add a lingering perk to their java, because it decreases the body's clearance of caffeine by 19%.[32]

While Lamisil is our first-line weapon against *T. rubrum*, the drug's performance against *Candida albicans* has been less impressive. Sporanox might possibly be the agent of choice for nail-unit infections caused by yeasts or molds, since it has the broadest spectrum of antifungal activity among our current systemic drugs. Taking advantage of itraconazole's persistence in the nail plate and bed, Janssen Pharmaceutica has been promoting a Sporanox "pulse regimen" for onychomycosis. In this regimen a patient takes a double dose of itraconazole (400 mg) each day for one week, then skips three weeks. Three or four "pulses"—that is, cycles of intermittent medication—constitute a course of treatment. The presumed advantage is cost-effectiveness, because the patient takes only one-half as much medication in pulse therapy as in the standard continuous therapy (200 mg itraconazole daily for twelve or sixteen weeks). A small early study of 49 patients with toenail onychomycosis reported mycological cure rates of 64% for a three-pulse itraconazole course and 72% for a four-pulse course.[33]

Like Sporanox, Lamisil can also be given in a pulse regimen, yet with either drug continuous therapy stands to put more medicine in the nail and to offer a better chance at cure. A big European trial whose results were published in 1999 has established that the continuous terbinafine regimens are significantly more effective than the itraconazole pulse regimens for toenail onychomycosis caused by dermatophytes. Enrollment in this trial was in fact limited to subjects with *Trichophyton* infections. Of the 496 patients recruited, 454 (91.5%) were afflicted by *T. rubrum*, and 42 (8.5%) by *T. mentagrophytes*. The

patients were randomly assigned to—and evenly
allotted between—four therapeutic schedules: to
twelve weeks of continuous terbinafine (250 mg
daily) or to sixteen weeks, or to three or to four
pulses of itraconazole (400 mg daily for one
week, then three weeks off). The trial's end point
was mycological cure (fungi-free nails), to be
determined at 72 weeks (upwards of a year and a
half) from the start of therapy. The final results
do not seem to need interpretation: 75.7% cured
by twelve weeks of continuous terbinafine and
80.8% cured by sixteen weeks, compared to
38.3% cured by three itraconazole pulses and
49.1% cured by four itraconazole pulses.[34]

I cannot say that I had even begun doing the
aforementioned pharmacological "homework" in
July 1999, at the time when I was completing my
own twelve-week Lamisil regimen. A naive and
trusting layperson, I simply marveled at the
changes those expensive white tablets had
wrought. New nail plate apparently free of fungus was already starting to grow out on that
second toe on my right foot, where the overt
symptoms of subungual onychomycosis had first

presented themselves a year before. Lamisil had now drawn a palpable horizontal ridge across the top of that nail. I could both see and feel the demarcation: it constituted an obvious front line in my struggle. Behind that line—on the proximal side—the nail plate and nail bed coming out of the matrix bore the fungicidal terbinafine molecules. In front of the line—on the distal side—lay the destructive occupying forces of the Red Fungus. As yet most of the toenail still belonged to the foe, but yes, there had been a very decided response to therapy. I later learned that proximal clearing after just several months on Lamisil is characteristic. Of course, the lion's share of the drug gets absorbed by the soft keratin of the newly-forming plate and bed in the matrix; comparatively little would seem to be absorbed by the hard distal plate.

As far as I could tell, my healthy toenails were not affected at all by terbinafine therapy; no lines of demarcation appeared on their dorsal surfaces. But after a few more days I started to see and feel an ominous little bulge moving forward on the big toenail of my right foot. That nail had remained morphologically normal, and I had not given it much thought. Now I realized

THE FRONT LINE AT TWELVE WEEKS

Second Toenail – Right Foot

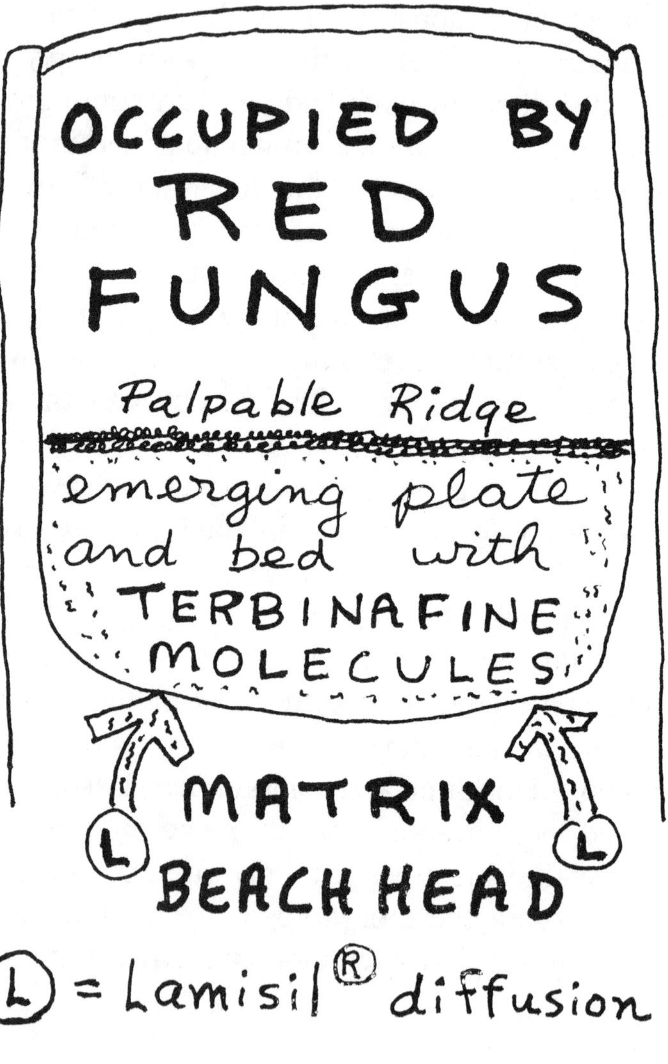

(L) = Lamisil® diffusion

that it had also been occupied by those disgusting dermatophytes, albeit surreptitiously, and that the slight bulge proximally simply represented a response to therapy.

Doctor P— seemed pleased when I saw him later in the month. While he ventured no prediction about the likelihood of an ultimate cure, he did sound optimistic: "You need to remember that the medicine remains in the nail, and it goes on working even after you stop taking it. I need to see you again in three months." In October 1999 I returned to Doctor P—'s office as instructed. "The nail is better," he observed, "but it is still involved. We have to wait and see whether the new nail will push out the involved portions. Come back and see me in four months."

This time I neglected to comply with that forceful invitation. I may have been unduly preoccupied with some other medical specialist, possibly with the dentist who does my root canals or with the orthopedist who handles my inflamed tendons and sprained ankles. In any event, I did not see Doctor P— again until May 2000, some seven months later. It was now ten months after I had completed my twelve-week Lamisil regimen.

On this occasion Doctor P— looked long and hard at the battlefield my toenails had become; he remained silent for a moment, then reached for a prescription pad and starting writing. "I want you to apply this lotion to those two nails once a day," he said, "right before you go to bed." He was referring to the diseased nails on my right foot, on the big toe and on the long-suffering second toe. "Try to raise the front edge of the nail up a little," he continued. "You want to get the lotion underneath the nail. I need to see you again in six months; but if those involved areas at the tip of the nail start to spread toward the base, I want you to come back sooner."

As Doctor P— exited the examining room, I looked at the prescription he had given me. It called for **Loprox® Lotion**. This is a dilute solution (0.77%) of **ciclopirox**, a broad-spectrum antibiotic which readily dispatches yeasts and bacteria as well as dermatophytes like *T. rubrum*. Loprox ought to be the right stuff for resistant cases of athlete's foot or jock itch, but Doctor P—'s sly insinuation that it might be made to penetrate through to the subungual regions was pure hooey. This topical formulation is not indicated for *tinea unguium*. I did not know this at the time; I have since come to realize that physicians who run out of meaningful therapeutic options may be strongly tempted to prescribe another drug which is unlikely to do harm or prove curative, yet which serves to create a simulation of ongoing therapy. In my case at least, the proper diagnosis in May 2000 would have been **TREATMENT FAILURE**, a frank admission which neither physicians nor pharmaceutical companies particularly relish. The Red Fungus may have retreated somewhat, but it was far from being destroyed. It remained entrenched in the distal nail bed and plate; any additional antifungal action from the Lamisil tablets I took in the preceding year was hardly to be expected.

No greater service can a medical writer perform for the public than an honest exposition of the limitations of an important yet imperfect pharmaceutical which has been fatuously ballyhooed in TV commercials. While Lamisil (terbinafine) can consistently eliminate 100% of the dermatophytes cultured in laboratory petri dishes, the pharmacokinetic circumstances of the body in general and of mycotic toenails in particular dictate that it will have a lower success rate in real-life cases of subungual onychomycosis. Let's briefly review some situations which spell for treatment failure; we will assume that the patient takes the medication as directed and that the nasty fungi are vulnerable to it. Yet nothing is going to happen if the ingested drug should fail to reach the affected toes. There may be a few patients whose livers are too efficient in metabo-lizing terbinafine; the upshot would be that not enough of the active agent gets into the blood-stream. With some patients the drug may get into the bloodstream, but then it never arrives at the embattled nail units because of compromised circulation to the digits. This situation can occur in diabetics and in persons with atherosclerosis or other vascular disorders. In my own case I could see that the drug was getting into the blood-stream, was arriving in the digits, and was dis-playing potent antifungal activity. I consequently began to suspect that the reason for my treatment failure was that I had not received an adequate regimen—viz., either not enough of the drug (inadequate dose) or a premature discontinuation of it (inadequate scheduling). Just because terbi-nafine tends to be retained in keratin, is it wise to discontinue therapy when we have reason to suspect that the nail unit still harbors viable fungi?

Roderick J. Hay, who has only good things to say about Lamisil, suggests "that terbinafine diffuses rapidly through the nail rather than being taken up into the proximal nail bed and growing out with the nail, as in the diffusion path of griseofulvin." Dr. Hay cites a small study (nine patients!) in which terbinafine was detected in distal toenail clippings "as early as three weeks after the start of therapy."[35] Well, maybe the drug does penetrate the distal nail plate in some patients, but I cannot say that I think this happened in my case. The rationale behind those quickie twelve-week regimens for Lamisil and Sporanox assumes both that our agent will diffuse into the distal plate from the distal nail bed, and that it will retain its antifungal activity for months on end. If either of these sanguine assumptions should prove unfounded, then it is unlikely that a short regimen will cure a long-established case of toenail onychomycosis.

To my mind, the reported terbinafine diffusion into the distal nail plate ought to be annotated with a question mark. There will probably be large variations between individual patients.

In general, we cannot anticipate that the dense mummified keratin of the distal plate will ever absorb a systemic antifungal as avidly as the fluid keratin in the matrix's living onychocytes. And the longer a dermatophyte infection persists in the nail unit, the less likely it is that distal diffusion will be efficient. These fungi eventually tend to form dense patches known as **dermatophytomas**; our antifungal drugs have difficulty penetrating these *nidi* (Latin, "nests") in much the same way that our cancer drugs fail to penetrate large solid tumors. And in advanced cases of subungual onychomycosis, the affected nail plate becomes thickened and is but loosely attached to the vascularized nail bed, especially in the lateral (side) grooves. This situation naturally impairs the diffusion of systemic agents from the bed into the plate.

But even if terbinafine only got into the matrix, it could still cure toenail onychomycosis if it retained full therapeutic activity for the year and a half that these nails require to grow out. Ah, there's the rub! While everybody agrees that this drug has a residual effect after discontinuance, nobody seems to know how long that effect lasts. I asked Doctor S—, a young podiatrist, for his opinion. "If you've just finished a course of Lamisil," he advised me, "you are protected for eight months. The reps say that the drug can be detected in the matrix a year later." The reps? Hang around doctors' offices long enough, and you'll eventually realize that those guys with black bags wandering in and out are not M.D.'s on their way to make house calls! They are simply "the reps"—i.e., sales representatives whose job it is to sell physicians on the merits of pricey new pharmaceuticals. I began to suspect that most practicing dermatologists and podiatrists did not have time to steep themselves in the pharmacological literature and were principally indebted to the reps' fast talk for their knowledge of Lamisil pharmacokinetics. No doubt traces of terbinafine can be detected in the matrix a year later, but this is not proof that you still have meaningful antifungal activity then, especially in the location where you are most likely to need it. Viz., down at the distal end of the toenails. That's where the fungi typically begin their inroads and where we would assume they are most deeply entrenched.

Anatomy of the
FAILED CAMPAIGN

distal
plate

proximal
Plate

*RF*RF*

*RF*RF*

MATRIX

distal
pincer

L = Lamisil® diffusion

RF = Red Fungus
entrenched

Failure of the author's
first terbinafine
offensive (April–July 1999)
has been attributed to
inadequate strength
in distal pincer.

Chapter Nine

Penlac™ Nail Lacquer

I seem to have gotten rather sloppy about keeping my appointments with Doctor P—. Almost eight months elapsed before I finally returned to his office, in January 2001. I had faithfully complied with his instructions for the use of Loprox® Lotion, applying it every night to the big toenail and the adjacent second toenail on my right foot. But now as Doctor P— surveyed the battlefield, he shook his head. "It's not getting any better," he said. "In fact, it may even be getting worse. Look—the big toenail on your left foot is also involved." *What?!?* Did he mean that the Red Fungus had actually advanced and now appeared to be winning the war? That left big toenail had never been mentioned before, and now it too was deemed a casualty. A painful silence ensued. Doctor P— sat down and started leafing through the voluminous handwritten notes in my file. Like me, he had gone to school back in the days when a computer was a bulky piece of equipment that took up an entire room and was used exclusively by mathematicians. He kept nothing electronically; from force of habit he recorded his clinical impressions, diagnoses, and prescriptions on a writing tablet, scribbling away with amazing speed at the same time he was explaining matters to his patients. After bending over my file for several minutes, he looked up optimistically, as though he might have found a way out of the therapeutic *cul-de-sac*. "There is a new drug I'd like to try," he said. "It's called Penlac, and it's only been on the market for a year. I want you to apply it once a day to those three nails. The box it comes in will contain additional printed instructions, which you need to read and follow carefully." He was already headed out the door: "I want to see you again in about five or six months."

Holding Doctor P—'s prescription like a beacon of hope, I trotted off to the low-price, fast-service drugstore around the corner. On this occasion the pharmacist did not ask me a single question; I paid $83.26 to fill my first Penlac prescription. At home I opened the little box and discovered a teeny-weeny bottle containing a mere 3.3 milliliters of antifungal lacquer. That's only 11% as much liquid as in a bottle of over-the-counter **Fungi-Nail®** (which contains 30 milliliters). I had previously purchased a bottle of Fungi-Nail from this same pharmacy for $17.64, and so I could arrive at an immediate price comparison. Fungi-Nail had cost me $0.59 per milliliter, Penlac $25.23. This new drug was packaged like a vial of the very finest French perfume—and priced to match! I handled the petite bottle most gingerly.

The active agent in Penlac is **ciclopirox**, the same antibiotic found in Loprox Lotion; yet these are substantially different products. Penlac has been especially formulated with a view to achieving agent penetration of mycotic nails. It consists of 8% ciclopirox, far more than in Loprox's 0.77% formulation. And when Penlac is applied to toenails or fingernails, the solvents in the lacquer (ethyl acetate and isopropyl alcohol) quickly evaporate, thus concentrating the active agent. The resulting film left on the nails will be upwards of 35% ciclopirox; and unless washed off, it will persist for many hours. Ciclopirox is a double-edged sword, killing fungal cells both by disrupting their outer membranes and by disabling the enzymes which sustain their metabolisms. The lacquer formulation is especially suited for the treatment of subungual onychomycosis because of its keratophilic properties. Like itraconazole and terbinafine, it is retained in nail keratin.[36]

As I pored over the lengthy directions that came in the Penlac box, I realized that debridement (removal) of the mycotic portions of the affected nails is an essential element in this topical therapy. Before an initial application of the lacquer, patients are advised to clip or file away "any loose nail or nail material." Then they are advised to apply Penlac "evenly over the entire nail" and insofar as possible "to the underside of the nail and to the skin beneath it." I later concluded that the manufacturer's counsel about "underside" application should be classified as wishful thinking or nebulous anatomy—if only it were true! Naturally you would want to put your Penlac in the distal and lateral nail grooves. Another counsel on the prescribing information proved equally unrealistic: "Allow lacquer to dry (approximately 30 seconds) before putting on socks or stockings." At best Penlac nail lacquer takes several minutes to dry completely; each time you open the bottle and expose it to air, it tends to get a little bit stickier and to take a little bit longer. The manufacturer recommends that you wait at least eight hours after each application "before taking a bath or shower." The reason is to allow that concentrated ciclopirox film as much time as possible to diffuse into the nail plate. Subsequent applications are simple: just paint the lacquer over the earlier coats and twiddle your thumbs while waiting for it to dry. Once a week you are supposed to remove the previous coats "with alcohol" and repeat the initial step of clipping or filing away any loose or obviously mycotic nail.[37]

I followed the aforementioned steps religiously. Now a seasoned veteran of the Toenail Fungus War, I appreciated the dual rationale for debridement. Viz., not only to remove the crumbly fungi-ridden matter, but also to roughen the surface of the harder and less involved nail plate so that the ciclopirox stood a better chance of sinking in. I decided to use those disposable nail files called "emery boards" for my weekly debridements. These are quite cheap (a package of ten for two bucks) and are typically found in the cosmetics department (not the pharmacy) of your drugstore or supermarket. By cutting an emery board into three pieces, I acquired a separate disposable file for each affected nail, and I did not have to worry about inadvertently transferring fungal elements from nail to nail via a contaminated metal file.

Once I had mastered the techniques of lacquer application and emery-board debridement, Penlac therapy quickly became a part of my daily routine. I felt like a fool for having to stop and paint my nails every night, but otherwise I experienced no ill effects. A few Penlac patients may have local reactions (inflammation, irritation, or itching) on the nearby skin, but it is unlikely that this topical agent will affect vital internal organs like the liver or the bone marrow. Unfortunately, when you have multiple nails to treat, you'll soon discover that after about a month the lacquer in the bottom of the bottle becomes so gummy as to be virtually unusable. As my weeks on therapy turned into months, I began to acquire a nice collection of three-quarters-empty Penlac bottles, each of which had retailed for $83.26 at my pharmacy. My average daily cost amounted to about $2.75—expensive, but still reasonable compared to Lamisil® tablets at ten dollars a pop. Is Penlac sufficiently efficacious to warrant all the bother?

Doctor P— gave me his professional opinion when I visited him in June 2001. "The nails are better," he said, "but the fungus is not eradicated." I could also see the improvement that five months of nightly Penlac applications had wrought. The distal portions (tips) of those three affected nails seemed to be clearing up—Penlac was certainly doing something! I had not noticed any change whatsoever with the two previous topical agents that Doctor P— had prescribed, the Oxistat and the Loprox. "You should continue using the Penlac for another six months," he told me. "If you should later need a second course of systemic therapy, the Penlac may improve the odds of success." *Six months more!* I felt condemned to march in place. "I guess it's like the lottery," I replied. "You just have to keep on playing until someday you win."

My three toenails were faithfully Pen-lacquered every night throughout the summer, not because I had any strong expectation of success, but because I had no alternative strategy. That second nail on my right foot continued to be a cause of concern. Yes, it was much clearer; but as far as I could tell, it had not grown so much as a millimeter for over a year. The last time I remembered seeing any outward movement in the nail plate was some two years before, after I had finished my twelve-week course of oral terbinafine. By September 2001 there was a definite indication of activity in that nail, but its significance was not immediately clear to me. A little bulge had developed in the proximal plate, right under the cuticle. Was that poor fungi-blasted nail finally starting to grow again? Within a few days the horrid truth revealed itself—this was not a return to vigor but **proximal subungual hyperkeratosis**. The pathological condition which I had noticed at the nail's tip in July 1998 was now presenting at the base. Penlac's success in suppressing distal disease had only served to mask the fact that the Red Fungus was alive and merrily multiplying in the nail matrix. Gradually the foe had amassed sufficient strength for renewed

FUNGAL COUNTERATTACK!

2nd Toenail, Rt. Foot, Sept. '01

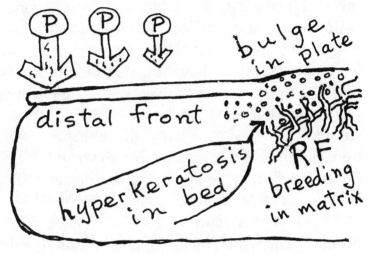

(P) = Penlac™ diffusion

RF = Red Fungus

---

author is lulled into
false sense of security by
Penlac successes on
distal front. Red Fungus
uses matrix breeding
ground to launch
massive assault on
proximal nail bed
and plate.

aggression. And now an inflammatory reaction
in the proximal nail bed was elevating the base of
the nail plate and loosening the fibrous bonds
which had held it in place. The thickened nail no
longer fit snugly in its lateral grooves but rode
high atop the toe. I thought that I could probably
pull it off with a pair of tweezers. The Grecian
noun **onycholysis** ("nail dissolution") can be
learnedly dropped to describe this unhappy situation; alternatively, the adjective **dystropic** ("not
flourishing") may be applied to the ravaged nail.
Both terms are as ominous as they are erudite.

In October I scurried back to Doctor P—'s
office. "There's a definite treatment failure with
this nail," he observed. Pressing tenderly against
it with his finger, he inquired: "Does that hurt?"
Pain is not a factor in the early stages of subungual onychomycosis.   Unlike athlete's foot or
jock itch, this disease does not cause physical
discomfort until it is far advanced, usually some
years after its inception. But thick dystrophic
nails which have risen out of the lateral grooves
are likely to cause problems for anyone who
wears shoes. The resulting mechanical irritation
of the surrounding skin (i.e., the nail grooves and
folds) tends to lead first to a painful inflammation

and then to secondary infections as bacteria and opportunistic fungi like *Candida albicans* arrive on the scene. I had seen vivid color photographs of severely dystrophic nails in textbooks, and I was beginning to suspect that pre-emptive ablation might be the best course of action. "Are we going to have to remove that nail?" I asked. Doctor P— gave me an admission which comes but rarely out of the mouths of veteran clinicians. "I don't know yet," he conceded.

Nine months of daily nail lacquering had served to enlighten me about the merits and limitations of Penlac. An advertisement in *People* magazine assures onychomycosis sufferers that "Penlac™ Targets the Problem—Not Your Whole Body." With Penlac "there's no need to worry about drug interactions, liver damage, or uncomfortable blood tests."[38] That much is true, and certainly we'd love to see a topical agent which could predictably cure all fungal infections of the nails. Unfortunately, Penlac by itself is a problematic weapon to use against subungual onychomycosis caused by *Trichophyton rubrum*, the most prevalent and most destructive toenail disease. This product may cure a *T. rubrum* infection which is just beginning underneath the tip (distal end) of the nail, but more advanced cases will continue to require an effective systemic drug like terbinafine (Lamisil® tablets) for any chance at cure. While ciclopirox lacquer has an unprecedented ability to penetrate and remain in the nail plate, there may be considerable variations between individuals with regard to the drug's diffusion through the plate into the nail bed. And that keratin-rich layer of the bed right beneath the plate tends to be a *hotbed* for the Red Fungus. To cure subungual onychomycosis due to *T. rubrum*, you must eliminate the dermatophytes from the nail bed as well as from the plate, and very often you also need to eliminate them from the nail matrix. Based on my own experience, I would say that ciclopirox lacquer applied to the dorsal plate has little or no ability to diffuse into the matrix, and that it should not be used as a sole agent in any case of onychomycosis where there is reason to suspect fungal activity in the matrix.

Some of the most illuminating studies of Penlac have been done in Germany, the country where this nail lacquer was first developed and marketed. One German study found that if less than 50% of the nail plate was involved with disease, "almost all nails recovered after six months of treatment." But apparent cures were not in evidence "if more than 50% of the nail area was affected at the onset of therapy."[39] The two American trials which led to FDA approval for Penlac also merit our attention: they enrolled a total of 465 patients with "distal subungual ony-chomycosis of the great toenail." That big toenail served as a "target nail"—i.e., the one which was used to assess therapeutic efficiency. At entry the eligible patients were deemed to have at least 25% of this nail involved, but no more than 60%. The intervention in both trials consisted of 48 weeks (about eleven months) of ciclopirox lacquer applied daily to the affected nails. Although almost all the patients improved on this regimen, there were only a modest number of verifiable cures in which the affected nails came to appear normal and were shown to be fungus-free by microscopic examination and laboratory culture. Richard K. Scher, a dermatologist at Columbia University, observes that "treatment success, defined as less than 10% involvement with negative mycology, was achieved by 13% of the patients in one study and 12% in the other."[40]

These two trials proved that Penlac is a safe and active agent for subungual onychomycosis caused by *T. rubrum.* Alas, they also demonstrated that even when we think we are dealing with disease confined to the distal portions of the nail unit, the tally of true cures with single-agent Penlac is not going to be very high. The manufacturer's prescribing information contains a statement in teeny-weeny print which sounds like a disclaimer: "A completely clear nail may not be achieved with use of this medication. In clinical studies less than 12% of patients were able to achieve either a clear or almost clear toenail."[41] Single-agent Penlac ought to give us a much higher success rate against those pesky fungal infections which usually remain on top of the nail plate—e.g., the white superficial onychomycosis which is caused by *T. mentagrophytes* and which mostly afflicts men, or the *Candida* infections of the fingernails which almost exclusively afflict women.

Chapter Ten

Using Our Weapons Better

A casual reader of the last two chapters may perhaps leap to the conclusion that the author is trying to debunk terbinafine hydrochloride tablets and ciclopirox nail lacquer. Nothing could be farther from my mind. I have come to praise these innovative pharmaceuticals. With Lamisil we have a well-tolerated systemic drug which can destroy the causative dermatophytes at extremely low concentrations. Penlac, a topical agent, can kill dermatophytes in the distal and lateral portions of the nail plate, sanctuaries which are not always reached by the diffusion of systemic drugs. Yet it is still no more appropriate to speak of a permanent "cure" for subungual onychomycosis than it would be to speak of a "cure" for diabetes, hypertension, or Parkinson's disease. The correct word is *management*. The advent of more effective systemic drugs and of keratophilic topical agents capable of penetrating the nail plate means that we now have weapons which can halt the relentless fungal dissolution of our toenails. Of course, this is not to say that effective management can be presently achieved without a considerable investment of time and money on the patient's part.

Those American physicians who treat onychomycosis are still learning how to use Lamisil and Penlac; unfortunately, the peripatetic sales reps sent out by the pharmaceutical companies may not be providing them with the highest level of instruction. With both these drugs, the standard regimens recommended by the manufacturer seem to have been designed more with a view to efficient marketing than to obtaining an optimal dose and scheduling in the individual case and highly variable circumstance.   Fingernails six weeks, toenails twelve weeks—the Lamisil recipes are easy to remember and go over well as sales pitches in the doc's office, now if only *Trichophyton rubrum* would cooperate!   We should not assume that terbinafine hydrochloride tablets are ineffective simply because a short regimen fails to produce a successful outcome.

In the United States ciclopirox nail lacquer has been promoted as a single-agent therapy for

T. rubrum subungual onychomycosis. Yet by itself Penlac is not going to halt disease progression in most cases; it would be the first choice only for those patients who cannot tolerate systemic drugs or whose disease seems confined to the distal half of the nail unit. A broader and more meaningful indication for keratophilic antifungal lacquers would be as supplemental agents used in conjunction with systemic therapy. Viz., a lacquer might be used concurrently (at the same time) with a systemic drug or soon after a course of systemic therapy. That systemic drug remains essential if we are to destroy the dermatophytes in the nail matrix and proximal nail bed, areas which even the new lacquers cannot penetrate very well. However, by using a lacquer on the dorsal surface of the nail plate, we might reduce the amount of systemic medication needed and obtain fungi-free nails much more rapidly. This optimistic scenario assumes that our topical agent will act synergetically with—enhance the effect of—our systemic drug, or at least that it will not prove antagonistic to (interfere with) the systemic drug's action.

Robert Baran of France is one onychomycosis expert who has been openly advocating combined therapy for "more severe cases presenting with lunula involvement and lateral nail disease, or with onycholysis, where the nail plate is no longer in contact with the subungual tissue."[42] Dr. Baran headed a small clinical trial which enrolled 147 patients suffering from "severe dermatophyte toenail onychomycosis with matrix area involvement." The trial's object was to test the usefulness of **amorolfine nail lacquer** as a supplemental agent in oral terbinafine therapy. Some of these patients received the standard Lamisil toenail regimen (250 mg daily for twelve weeks); others received the same Lamisil regimen, but also applied amorolfine lacquer to their affected nails once a week for fifteen months. The results which Dr. Baran published in the *British Journal of Dermatology* in October 2001 revealed a clear advantage for the combined therapy. While only 37.5% of the patients receiving the standard oral regimen had achieved "mycological and clinical cure" a year and a half later, 72.3% of those who also used the nail lacquer had done so.[43]

Amorolfine nail lacquer, marketed in England and many other countries under the brand name **Loceryl**, has not been available in the United

States. American onychomycosis sufferers would therefore be greatly benefited if somebody would do a large clinical trial which would tell us conclusively whether ciclopirox nail lacquer should—or should not—be used concurrently with oral terbinafine. Since Penlac kills fungal cells by different mechanisms from Lamisil, we might hope that the concurrent use of these agents would produce a decidedly synergetic effect— viz., that the two drugs together would do a better job than either one alone. Of course, there is no way of confirming this hypothesis without a well-designed trial with long-term follow-up. The August 2000 edition of the Penlac prescribing information advises against any concurrent therapy, observing that "no studies have been conducted to determine whether ciclopirox might reduce the effectiveness of systemic antifungal agents."[44] This blanket statement is not altogether appropriate, for at least one German study had previously reported an impressive 88% cure rate in toenail onychomycosis when ciclopirox nail lacquer was used concurrently with intermittent itraconazole (the Sporanox pulse regimen).[45]

Few politicians would dare to do such a transparent sidestepping of critical issues as that which we find in the Penlac prescribing information. How often must a suffering patient apply the lacquer, and how long must he stay on the tedious routine? The drug's manufacturer just says "daily," a recommendation perhaps more strongly related to an urge to profitability than to the existing clinical data. Daily application of Penlac for many months on end would seem to represent excessive dose and scheduling. The reason is that both the amorolfine and ciclopirox lacquers quickly achieve a steady-state concentration of the agent in the nail plate; after a month or two of daily use, a less frequent scheduling— say, one application a week—may well suffice to maintain that concentration and presumably any therapeutic benefits to be had. A large trial done at the Technical University of Dresden and other German institutions enrolled 1,222 onychomycosis patients with a view to determining the optimal frequency of ciclopirox lacquer application. Patients were divided into four groups with different schedules: once a week, twice a week, three times a week, four-to-seven times a week. The trial lasted six months. At the end of the first month, the percentage of patients with "improved symptoms" was noticeably higher in the group applying the lacquer twice a week (60% improved) and in the groups applying it three or more times a week (63% improved) than in the group which applied it only once a week (51% improved). However, the German researchers discovered that "after three months of treatment, these differences all leveled to nearly 70%, independent of treatment frequency. This percentage of treatment success did not change towards the end of the study." The scheduling recommendation which these researchers published would certainly save American Penlac patients a bundle of money and a mountain of aggravation. Apply the lacquer three times a week for the first month, the Germans urge, "to quickly reach an ungual penetration of ciclopirox and a persistent steady-state concentration." For the second month "twice weekly application seems to be sufficient." Thereafter "the compound should be applied at least once weekly to ensure the antifungal properties."[46] The optimal frequency of application no doubt needs to be verified by additional trials, as does the broader question of treatment duration. How long should a patient stay on Penlac? A year? Two years? Indefinitely? Just because this agent carries virtually no risk of systemic toxicity, there can still be no justification for prescribing it above and beyond any reasonable expectation of therapeutic benefit.

The state of affairs with the recommended Lamisil regimens stands in sharp contrast to Penlac. In this instance an unbiased front-line observer like myself feels duty-bound to report his suspicions of *inadequate* dose and scheduling. Are patients on these regimens really getting enough of the drug—and staying medicated for enough time—to achieve the maximum success rates? Assuming that the ingested terbinafine is reaching the nail unit and that the dermatophytes have not developed resistance to it, why couldn't we cure almost all onychomycosis cases simply by appropriately escalating the dose and/or lengthening the scheduling? The main stumbling block to this more flexible strategy has less to do with pharmacokinetics than with fears of litigation. Unlike ciclopirox nail lacquer, oral terbinafine is an agent which may cause serious side effects in a very few patients. And if this drug is given to tens of millions, sooner or later it will be inadvertently or recklessly prescribed for a small number of patients with liver disease or kidney dysfunction, with possibly fatal consequences. The risk of mishaps may also be presumed to increase with higher dosage levels and lengthier courses of treatment. Thus while we are given the manufacturer's leave to pour on the Penlac all the days of our lives, the Lamisil prescribing information reads like a long-winded *caveat emptor* (you can't say you weren't warned!) and says not a word about adjusting the dose or the scheduling. Toenails twelve weeks, 250 mg daily—this quickie low-dose recipe is offered as a commandment. The risk of toxicity is certainly minimized, the treatment's brevity sounds appealing, and the product liability lawyers haven't got a thing to work with.

Unfortunately, in my own case I had already experienced treatment failure on the twelve-week Lamisil regimen in 1999; thus I had no reason to expect that it would vanquish the more entrenched dermatophyte infection that I was facing in the autumn of 2001. And now my dermatologist Doctor P— seemed to be coming down with a bad case of defeatism (they call this mind-set **therapeutic nihilism** in medical circles). "You have already had the best available therapy," he

told me. "Even when a patient has a good response to Lamisil, the problem usually comes
back in a year or two. The dermatology profess-
ors are simply publishing a lot of stuff to justify
their existence. Combined therapy with terbinafine and itraconazole, things like that, all of
which add up to terrible liver toxicity." Was
Doctor P— about to abandon my fight and
sheepishly urge submission to the will of God?
My years in the Army had taught me not to be
demoralized by temporary setbacks, at least not
when there were weapons at hand to use against
the foe. For heaven's sake, this enemy was a
stupid vulnerable microorganism, not pancreatic
cancer or a brain tumor. But I had seen how that
humble Red Fungus had somehow managed to
turn the second toenail on my right foot into a
dystrophic Hamburger Hill, and I was increasingly anxious to save my two big toenails from
a similar fate. Yes, those nails had long since
assumed the sickly opaque coloration which bespeaks early-stage subungual onychomycosis; but
as yet they were morphologically normal, and
they continued to grow out. Could not they be
rescued? "I'd like to treat this problem aggressively," I told Doctor P—, "let's hit the fungus

with everything we've got." He was already slipping out the door of the examining room. Every fiber in my being, conditioning by military training and too many war movies, resounded to a single internal command: *Attack! Attack! Attack!*

I promptly retreated to a medical library, where I pounced on the dermatology journals with a passion. Did somebody have a better strategy for using oral terbinafine? In the July 2000 issue of *Archives of Dermatology*, I found a brief document which suited my purposes to a T. The Miami Beach dermatologists Nardo Zaias and Gerbert Rebell had written this journal to express their opinion that "the tested regimens for the treatment of onychomycosis are not optimal and are misleading with respect to efficacy." Do tell! The emperor has no clothes! Doctors Zaias and Rebell observed that the precise diffusion paths of terbinafine and itraconazole have yet to be defined. We really do not know how much of the orally administered drug "enters the nail bed and overlying nail plate through the entire area of the nail bed," or how much "is incorporated into these structures in their individual matrix regions and then moves distally." Of course, if our drug principally goes into the matrix and then slowly moves out with the new nail plate, then short regimens could well be ineffective, particularly if the agent's "fungistatic or fungicidal properties" wear off before "the time required to replace the entire toenail by normal growth."

The terbinafine regimen that Zaias and Rebell had been using in their practice was a far cry from the standard twelve-week course. They opted instead for low-dose intermittent (pulse) administration whereby toenail onychomycosis patients with culture-proven *T. rubrum* nail bed involvement took oral terbinafine (250 mg daily) for only one week of each month. But then their patients stayed on therapy "for eleven or more months, until the mycotic nail bed had been completely replaced by new nonmycotic nail bed." Zaias and Rebell were sticklers for detail. Before treatment they put a little notch in a target nail to establish the extent of the underlying disease, and they checked their patients every month to verify an ongoing response to therapy. Any patient whose disease spread proximally during treatment was "removed from the study." Just two of the twenty patients Zaias and Rebell kept tabs on experienced treatment failure; the others were eventually "recorded as cures," based both on clinical observation and on the absence of fungi as demonstrated by microscopy and laboratory culture. Zaias and Rebell pointed out that their 90% cure rate "exceeds those reported in the large studies."[47]

I found this optimistic report wonderfully refreshing after the gloom-and-doom assessment that Doctor P— seemed to be giving me on my last office visit. If a patient is responding to Lamisil and the drug is causing no side effects, why discontinue it before you have a verifiable cure? I concluded that prolonged terbinafine pulse therapy ought to be the right approach to save my big toenails. Intermittent administration should suffice because the drug exerts a residual action, even after a modest seven-tablet pulse; moreover, it should give my liver and my pocket-book a little time off to recuperate. But I wondered whether the overall dose in the Zaias and Rebell regimen might be too low to guarantee success; after all I had failed the twelve-week regimen, and what they had done was simply to give the standard dose over a period of some twelve months instead of twelve weeks. While I applauded the lengthened scheduling, I felt that a modest dose escalation was surely indicated in my case. For many years I had been an avid follower of new developments in cancer medicine, and of course I was familiar with the terribly complicated manipulations of drug dosage and scheduling that oncologists (the cancer chemotherapy doctors) are constantly making in hopes of obtaining improved survival rates. Cooking up a better recipe for Lamisil tablets looked like child's play. In five minutes I had done the task to my satisfaction. I wanted to begin with what the oncologists call a **loading dose**—viz., a larger initial dose of the drug given with a view to starting a therapeutic response. This would be followed by periodic cycles (pulses) of a **maintenance dose**—viz., smaller doses given at regular intervals to maintain the response. With my pocket calculator I did a hasty reckoning. Thirty Lamisil tablets up front for one-month continuous therapy (that would be my loading dose), to be followed by ten tablets a month for the ensuing year (that would be my long-term pulse therapy for maintenance). Let's see—assuming the tablets cost about ten dollars each, that would be about $300 for the first month, then about $100 per month for the ensuing year, or about $1,500 all told for the medication. This cost projection actually struck me as reasonable. The final cost of letting the Red Fungus destroy those big toenails, and of having to engage a podiatrist later to extract the stumps, might prove to be far higher, whether measured in dollars and cents or in terms of physical pain and psychological anguish.

When I saw Doctor P— again, he listened politely to the details of my proposed regimen. Then he assumed the posture of authority. "If the nail plate is completely involved," he said, "what they do is to give sixteen weeks of Lamisil." Who were "they" I wondered, and where was Doctor P— getting his facts? I suspected those fast-talking sales reps, but there was little I could do about it. Doctor P— held the prescription pad, not I, and he was now handing me a prescription for a two-month supply of Lamisil tablets. "You need to come back in two months," he said. Unhappy, I ventured a modest protest: "I don't think it is advisable to discontinue treatment altogether before the fungus is destroyed. Can I go on the pulse regimen after I finish the sixteen weeks?" Doctor P— answered as he headed out the door: "We'll talk about that the next time."

Well, if I did not yet have my maintenance therapy, at least I had a cornucopia of a loading dose: Doctor P— proposed to give me 120 tablets up front! Because I was purchasing the drug in sixty-tablet increments, the bill for that cherished prescription came to a mere $559, or $9.32 per tablet. Two months later—in December 2001—I had finished the first sixty tablets, but my three involved toenails looked much the same. "Go ahead and refill the prescription," advised Doctor P—. Another $559 down the drain, and still no commitment from him about long-term mainte-nance!

I completed the sixteen-week regimen in February 2002. Doctor P— did not sound overly optimistic as he glanced at my toenails: "It doesn't look like you've absorbed enough of the drug." In truth, there had as yet been few dis-cernable changes to the affected nails, but my confidence in Lamisil therapy remained high because I knew that clinical observations early on cannot always gauge this drug's ultimate effects. And whatever reservations Doctor P— may have privately held about prescribing Lamisil beyond the manufacturer's published recommendations, he had decided to bend the rules just a tad. The prescription he now handed me called for four-teen (14) additional Lamisil tablets. "I want you to wait three weeks," he told me, "then take a tablet a day for one week. Then wait another three weeks and repeat the process." Hurrah! So Doctor P— was letting me have my pulse therapy as maintenance, though not quite at the ten-tablet dose level I wanted and definitely not without strings attached. The annotation *No refills* was underscored at the bottom of the prescription, by way of emphasizing that he wanted to monitor my response to treatment and my state of health somewhat more closely than he had in the past.

On a per-pill basis the pharmacy around the corner charged me noticeably more to fill this odd-lot prescription: $156.53 or exactly $11.18 per Lamisil tablet. At the moment, however, I was less concerned with the rapidly escalating cost of therapy than with the progressive deterioration of the dystrophic second toenail on my right foot. The tip of the nail had begun to crumble away since I discontinued the Penlac lacquer some four months earlier. I now hastened to seek counsel from my podiatrist friend Doctor S—. "It's too soon to remove this nail," he told me. "We try to avoid removing toenails because extraction always disrupts the nail unit and it carries a risk of infection. The old dystrophic nail plate will eventually fall or peel off, much like an old snake skin. In the meantime you might want to go back to using Penlac." I asked Doctor S— whether he thought the Penlac would in any way interfere with the Lamisil. He shook his head: "The drugs work by different mechanisms. The Penlac won't hurt, and it should help. You could put the Penlac on all three affected nails, but if you have to choose, certainly on that dystrophic second nail."

I knew that Doctor S—'s upbeat advice was racing ahead of any mature clinical trials whose data might establish the concurrent use of Penlac and Lamisil. So I decided to hedge my bets. I felt that I had nothing to lose by trying concurrent Penlac on the second toenail; I doubted that Lamisil alone would help this nail much, because its matrix had presumably been scarred by chronic infection, and because its plate no longer had the closest contact with the nail bed. In the case of the big toenails, I believed that the vascular diffusion pathways into the matrices and the nail beds should be intact, and that the newly-forming nail plates would surely incorporate any terbinafine molecules which reached the toes. Lamisil alone ought to defeat the Red Fungus on these two larger battlefields. I did not wish to compromise a battle plan with a good probability of success by employing a secondary weapon whose role in this circumstance had not been precisely defined. Frankly, it also occurred to me that I now enjoyed a splendid opportunity to observe and report the therapeutic actions of our two best onychomycosis agents. Was there not a vast reading public which hungered for a book entitled *Mein Nagelkampf,* and were not my toenails a representative microcosm of this disease? That second toenail was so far advanced in dissolution that I had contemplated its removal; the big toenails, while involved throughout, represented a much earlier stage of pathology.

I decided to monitor my response to treatment more closely than I had with the abortive Lamisil campaign of 1999 and the ill-fated Penlac offensive of 2001. Every week I tried to take time to sit in bright sunlight and inspect the affected nails under a magnifying glass. That second toenail looked terrible; at least the nightly Penlac applications and the weekly debridements were getting rid of the crumbling distal portions of the plate, but the proximal plate retained a deep yellow coloration suggestive of densely intertwined fungal hyphae. Things looked more promising on the Big Toenail Front, where oral terbinafine was the sole weapon being employed. By March 2002 I could see a definite improvement in the proximal regions; that sickly opaque coloration which indicates nail bed involvement was starting to give way to a more pinkish tone. After I completed my two pulse doses, I checked back with Doctor P—. "Any response to Lamisil always begins proximally," he said. "I've never had a patient where the response began distally." He seemed satisfied with my progress; and he handed me a prescription for another fourteen tablets, clearly marked "no refills." In other words, come back and see the doc when you need some more!

The lines of demarcation on those big toenails were becoming ever more pronounced. Even an untrained layperson could see the striking difference between the proximal regions which had been liberated from the Red Fungus, and the distal regions still in the grip of the foe. Week by week the front on both nails moved inexorably forward, toward the tips. I assumed that what I

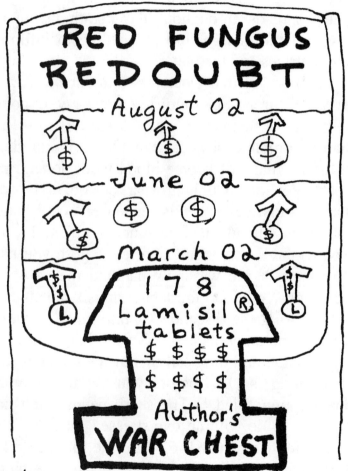

was observing resulted from effective antifungal action on the infected nail beds. *T. rubrum* typically spreads throughout the keratinous upper layer of the beds before proceeding to infiltrate the matrices and the plates.

When I visited Doctor P— in June 2002, he seemed surprisingly indifferent to my ongoing response to therapy. "When is the last time you had a complete physical exam?" he inquired. I told him that I had some blood work done at the local Veterans Clinic a year before. He was hardly satisfied with this response: "Well, since you have already had so much Lamisil, I want you to have a liver function test before you take any more." He was now handing me two prescriptions, one for fourteen Lamisil tablets and one bearing the direction *hepatic panel*. "Don't forget," he admonished. "Get the lab work done right away, and then call this office to check that everything is O.K. before you get that Lamisil prescription filled." The sharp pangs I felt had nothing to do with an overstressed liver: $75 for the office visit and $156.53 for the fourteen pills, to which would now be added $55 for the blood test. Heck! If yer liver don't fail, yer piggy bank sure will!

Doctor P— was all smiles when I visited him in August. "Your liver function test came back fine," he told me, "everything perfectly normal." The dual specters of surreptitious hepatotoxicity and ensuing malpractice litigation appeared to have been banished. Doctor P— sounded truly optimistic for the first time in several years. "The more experience we have with Lamisil," he opined, "the more we realize that our fears of toxicity were exaggerated. It is a very safe drug." On this occasion he gave me a prescription for twenty-one (21) Lamisil tablets, enough for three pulse doses. My big toenails now looked almost clear, except for thin rims of discoloration at their tips. Even that fungi-blasted second nail had shown a few signs of outward growth. Total victory over the Red Fungus seemed imminent. Alas, I hardly anticipated the foe's next move.

During my weekly nail inspections in sun-light, I had noticed a curious phenomenon: a thin white streak was becoming ever more visible on the dorsal (top) surface of the right big toenail. This streak began at the nail's tip (free edge) and descended like a falling arrow toward the cuticle, seemingly disappearing in the middle of the plate. At first I thought nothing of it, but by September it had gotten bigger and cried out for an explanation. What was it? I found the appalling answer in a new book entitled *Nagelmykosen* from the pen of Isaak Effendy, a dermatologist in Bielefeld, Germany. There it was on page 44, a splendid color illustration of a big toenail with a white streak starting at the tip and running longitudinally down to the cuticle. Dr. Effendy called this particular presentation a **Streifenbefall**—probably a more memorable term than the literal English translation, which is "attack along the line."[48] *Streifenbefälle* are almost certainly more common on the big toenails than on their neighbors. The mechanism of disease is easy to understand: *T. rubrum* embeds itself in a tiny groove in the ventral nail plate, which could be either a crack produced by trauma or a naturally occurring seam. Over a period of time the Red Fungus enlarges that groove and expands upward in the plate, eventually producing a palpable ridge on top. In my case the *Streifenbefall* was still small and hardly the stuff of which textbook illustrations are made. But the fact that it had arisen during my protracted Lamisil therapy can serve as a caution. However effective oral terbinafine may be in diffusing into the nail matrix and the

STREIFENBEFALL
(Right Big Toenail, Sept. '02)

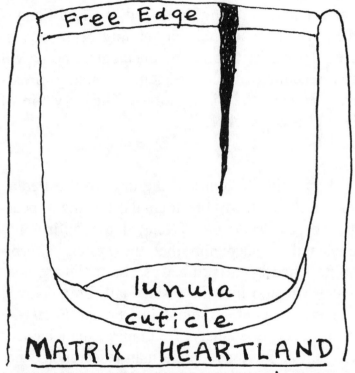

Free Edge

lunula

cuticle

MATRIX HEARTLAND

The Red Fungus survives Lamisil® bombardment by entrenchment in nail plate crevice; later resumes march toward the matrix.

proximal nail bed, this agent does not readily achieve fungitoxic concentrations against dermatophytes which have burrowed into the distal nail plate. Far from being destroyed, the Red Fungus in my right big toenail had simply been sequestered during the terbinafine onslaught, and now it was resuming its aggression, tunneling proximally toward the vital matrix. The very life of the nail was at stake!

I had hitherto resisted the urge to use Penlac concurrently on my big toenails; but the appearance of a *Streifenbefall* tended to confirm my longstanding suspicion that the systemic terbinafine I had been taking was not achieving adequate diffusion into the distal nail unit. Now I decided to launch an immediate Penlac *Blitzkrieg* on those big toenails. If ciclopirox nail lacquer was half as good as the German researchers said, it ought to be able to halt this intraungual subversion in short order. Taking a cue from Dr. Baran and the Germans, I applied Penlac daily only for six weeks; thereafter I switched to thrice-weekly application. That cut my expense and aggravation roughly in half, while guaranteeing a potent steady-state concentration of ciclopirox in the nail plate. In any event, the battle developed exactly as I had hoped. What systemic terbinafine had been unable to do, the topical agent quickly accomplished. After some three weeks of Penlacquering, I could no longer discern the faintest trace of the *Streifenbefall*. That thin white streak had vanished; presumably the ciclopirox had seeped down into the nail crevice and routed those disgusting dermatophytes.

By the beginning of October 2002, the areas of suspicious discoloration on my big toenails were limited to the extreme distal corners. And these pockets of resistance soon yielded to my aggressive two-pronged offensive, whereby the ciclopirox molecules came down through the dorsal plate at the same time the terbinafine forces were filtering upwards from the nail bed. By the end of October those big toenails looked perfectly healthy. Even with a magnifying glass I could not detect any obvious signs of fungal activity, but of course I wanted an opinion from someone who had considerable clinical experience with toenail onychomycoses. "Do I have a cure yet?" I asked my podiatrist friend Doctor S—. "Not quite," he answered. "The big toenails do look good, but portions of that second toenail on your right foot need to be trimmed. If you want to obtain the maximum benefit from Penlac, you have to have the affected nails professionally debrided every so often." Doctor S— deftly stripped away the mycotic lateral portions of that second toenail, and then gently shaved the distal tips of my big toenails. The operation took a mere ten minutes and was virtually painless.

My dermatologist Doctor P— constituted the acid test insofar as a clinical judgment might be concerned. With his thirty years of experience eyeballing dermatological problems, he ought to be able to recognize mycoticly involved toenails as well as anybody in town. But when I visited him in the first week of November 2002, he hardly said hello, just bent over and took a little scraping from the tip of one of my big toenails. He then left the examining room; when he returned twenty minutes later, he did not mince words. "You don't need any more Lamisil," he said emphatically, with a faint aura of triumph. Was I really cured? After fighting the Red Fungus for almost four years, could I finally claim victory? Ever cautious, Doctor P— made no sweeping pronouncements about the status of my

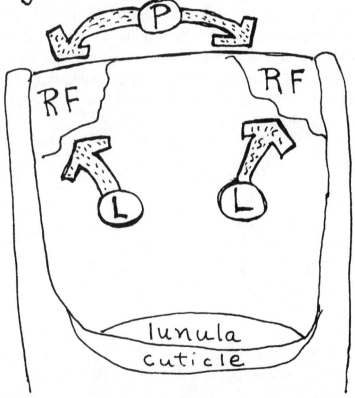

MOPPING UP THE RESISTANCE
Big Toenail Front, Oct. '02

RF = Encircled pockets of RED FUNGUS

(L) = Lamisil® upward diffusion

(P) = Penlac™ downward diffusion

toenails, but for once he did not suggest a temporal framework for my next appointment. "Come back if you see any signs of recurrent activity on those toenails," he advised me as he moved on to another patient. Thus the matter of a return visit had been left entirely to my discretion. In the imprecise world of toenail fungus medicine, that particular detail was as much of a victory parade as I could hope for.

Chapter Eleven

Toenail Surgery:
The Scorched-Earth Strategies

F or generations—indeed, up until the mid-1990s—virtually all Americans who suffered from subungual onychomycosis eventually became candidates for surgery. The available topical antifungals did nothing to slow dermatophyte proliferation in the nail bed and matrix; and griseofulvin, the old systemic drug, usually proved ineffective. By the year 2000 those innovative pharmaceuticals Lamisil® tablets and Penlac™ nail lacquer held out the promise of healthy toenails; it would surely be fulfilled if patients would seek treatment at the first sign of this disease, and if physicians would prescribe these products in a sophisticated fashion tailored to the individual case. Unfortunately, even assuming these prerequisites are met, an efficacious course of therapy with either agent, or with both, requires a great deal of time and meticulous attention to detail; and at present it may well cost several thousand dollars before its completion. Perhaps only a minority of sufferers are enlightened about nail anatomy and the infectious process, or sufficiently persevering to endure the long struggle for the hardly inevitable cure. As a consequence, toenail surgery to relieve the symptoms of advanced disease will continue to be necessary in many cases.

The Philadelphia podiatrist Warren S. Joseph reminds us that thickened dystrophic toenails can lead to serious complications in persons who have diabetes or "peripheral vascular disease" (i.e., poor circulation in the extremities). Reduced sensation or circulation in the toes will predispose the onychomycosis sufferer to local infections and ulcerations, and in the worst scenario, to gangrene. "Because of the sensory neuropathy," Dr. Joseph cautions, "the patient may be unaware of the thickness or length of the toenail until the nail has damaged adjacent skin, potentiating a deep infection. With poor perfusion to the digits, ulcerations and wounds heal with difficulty."[49] Elderly or infirm patients have a noticeably higher risk for these complications.

Younger persons with adequate sensation and circulation in their toes probably will not fall prey to infections and ulcerations; but the more active they are, the more likely they are to be troubled by pain and social embarrassment. In late-stage subungual onychomycosis, the toenails may look disgusting, and searching for a comfortable pair of shoes tends to become an endless Grail quest.

Anyone with thickened mycotic toenails stands to benefit from a visit to a podiatrist. The simplest approach in these cases is **debridement**, the mechanical reduction of a toenail's bulk. What the podiatrist can do in a few minutes will be much more satisfactory than anything the patient can accomplish by himself. A stainless steel instrument called a "nail nipper" is employed to shave off most of the thickened nail plate. An electric drill with a rotating bur at the end is then used to smooth the dorsal surface of the remaining plate. We must emphasize that debridement does not cure subungual onychomycosis; it is a palliative measure which lessens pain, makes shoes fit more comfortably, and reduces the risk of secondary infections and ulcerations. But patients with thick dystrophic toenails who hope to be cured by Lamisil tablets or by Penlac would be well advised to undergo debridement before beginning drug therapy: the removal of most of the mycotic nail plate probably betters the odds of a favorable outcome.

The surgical procedure which does cure subungual onychomycosis is called **avulsion and matricectomy**. This option of last resort offers a more permanent solution than pharmaceuticals: the nail plate, the bed, and the matrix are ablated (i.e., totally removed). If there is no toenail, there can be no toenail fungus. A scorched-earth strategy never fails to stop the invader! And compared to repeated courses of systemic terbinafine, it is cheap and fast, if necessarily entailing more physical and psychological discomfort. The procedure can be accomplished during one visit to a podiatrist's office.

The involved toe is first desensitized by injecting a local anesthetic, usually lidocaine, at several sites around the digit. After the anesthetic takes effect, a flexible tourniquet is applied at the base of the toe, so as to control bleeding. The nail plate is loosened by inserting a flat metal spatula under the distal tip (the free edge) and pushing forward gently but firmly. This creates a cleavage between the plate and the bed. The spatula is next inserted under the cuticle, the other point of strong attachment between the plate and the surrounding tissues. Once these several bonds holding the plate in place have been destroyed, it can be avulsed (pulled away) with a gentle rolling motion. Matricectomy, the second half of the procedure, is accomplished by applying a concentrated solution of phenol to the exposed matrix. This toxic chemical produces permanent ablation in a few seconds; afterwards the matrix and the bed are flushed with alcohol to dilute and wash away the traces of phenol.

A patient who has just undergone avulsion and matricectomy of the hallux (big toe) can walk out of the podiatrist's office unaided, but may be hampered in driving a car by the cumbersome dressing put on the toe. This dressing needs to be both bulky and absorbent, so as to cushion the wound from impact and to absorb the serous discharge. A mild narcotic formulation featuring codeine or oxycodone, similar to those prescribed after tooth extractions, normally suffices for pain control in the immediate postoperative period. For the first few days after surgery, the patient ought to keep the affected foot elevated as much as possible, with a view to minimizing swelling and promoting drainage. Stuart J. Salasche, an Arizona dermatologist, advises that "the dressing should be changed daily until exudation has stopped and pain abated. If the dressing is not changed frequently, the serosanguineous or sero-purulent material may act as media for bacteria." The wound can be cleaned with a dilute solution of hydrogen peroxide, but should otherwise be kept dry. Dr. Salasche reminds nail surgery patients who change their own dressings that the "securing adhesive tape must not be placed completely around the digit because it may act as a constricting band if swelling occurs."[50]

Full recovery from avulsion and matricectomy can take six weeks or more. Ultimately, the healing nail bed assumes a leathery consistency; the tough new skin mimics the missing nail plate and provides at least some protection for the digit. Female patients sometimes apply nail polish to the healed bed, making the absence of a plate less obvious. Of course, that plate is gone for good, because the nail-forming onychocytes in the matrix have been destroyed by the phenol application.

Avulsion without matricectomy is a surgical option for advanced subungual onychomycosis which leaves open the possibility of nail regrowth. After the nail is removed, a systemic antifungal like terbinafine or itraconazole can almost always eradicate the dermatophyte infection. Unfortunately, the reappearance of a functional and cosmetically appealing toenail is much less certain: the plate may need a year or two to grow back, and it may have significant imperfections. Because the regrowing plate is no longer following the track of an existing plate, it may tend to painfully embed itself in the distal nail bed or in the lateral nail folds. Robert Baran and his colleagues recommend that "the patient use a prosthetic nail on the regrowing plate so that the width of the nail bed is maintained and subsequent ingrowth is avoided."[51]

The **chemical dissolution** of dystrophic nail plates is a bloodless alternative to avulsion; it would be indicated in patients likely to experience complications after toenail surgery (e.g., the elderly and persons with diabetes or peripheral vascular disease). Sometimes referred to as a "chemical avulsion," this procedure is simple and inexpensive, although time-consuming for the physician and inconveniently messy for the patient. A thick ointment consisting of urea and white petroleum jelly is put on the affected nails, while the surrounding healthy skin is protected by an adhesive dressing. The treated toenails are then wrapped; they must remain occluded (covered up) for about a week. During this time the urea, a water-soluble keratolytic compound, penetrates and softens the mycotic nail plates. Afterwards these plates can usually be lifted off without anesthesia and without risk of hemorrhage or infection.[52] Other advantages of urea ointment include the ability to treat multiple nails at the same time and to repeat the procedure as often as needed. A noticeable disadvantage is the unpleasant odor which accompanies urea keratolysis. The olfactory insult is intensified by the fact that the patient cannot bathe his feet during the week-long occlusion. By itself a chemical avulsion cannot guarantee the removal of all portions of the nail plate, and it does nothing to combat any dermatophytes which may be lurking in the matrix.

Chapter Twelve

Keeping the Enemy at Bay

A thlete's foot and toenail fungus can be viewed as microbiology's sardonic retribution for the evils of colonialism. We may be reasonably certain that George Washington and Abraham Lincoln did not suffer from these now prevalent dermatomycoses. Nobody did during the eighteenth and nineteenth centuries. The first well-documented cases of athlete's foot in the United States did not occur until the 1920s. How did the current epidemic come to pass? The blame lies with those smug representatives of Western civilization, mainly soldiers and missionaries, who brought the benefits of Christianity and cannons to certain undeveloped regions in Africa and Asia. While *Trichophyton rubrum* was endemic in these warm humid climates, the native inhabitants were not troubled. They may have carried this pernicious dermatophyte on their feet, yet they did not develop disease, possibly because they had developed resistance to it over the course of thousands of years. Equally important, these native Africans and Asians either went barefoot or opted for loose sandal-type footwear. The Europeans and Americans who marched into their homelands had never encountered *T. rubrum* before; they had less resistance to it, and even on the sultriest days they wore combat boots or tight-laced shoes, occlusive leather footwear which might as well have been specially designed for dermatophyte incubation. And these silly imperialists actually looked down on the barefoot natives! Little did they know that their descendants would pay a terrible price for their arrogant assumption of cultural superiority.

Today the humble *T. rubrum* continues to mock the peculiarly Occidental faith that science and technology must inevitably triumph over nature. If you have once suffered from athlete's foot or toenail fungus, how do you prevent a recurrence of disease? Unfortunately, we have no simple reliable prophylaxis for *tinea pedis* and *tinea unguium*, any more than we have a simple reliable prophylaxis for colon cancer or Alzheimer's disease. To banish *T. rubrum* for good, we will first need to discover the secrets behind its remarkable ability to persist in the environment and on human feet. In the meantime there is no shortage of suggestions from eminent dermatologists and podiatrists on ways to reduce the frequency and severity of these infections. The proposed strategies ought to keep your toes and toenails from being absolutely devastated by the Red Fungus: they are therefore worth being repeated here, though the author must add the prudent caveat that we have as yet no hard data on their actual level of effectiveness.

Occlusive footwear is the Original Sin of *tinea* sufferers. *The Merck Manual*, a reference book found in doctors' offices, offers the obvious counsel that "many patients even benefit from going barefoot."[53] True enough, but more practical for beachcombers than city dwellers! The dermatologist Thomas P. Habif and his colleagues at the Dartmouth Medical School are somewhat mindful of feasibility issues in their recent textbook on skin diseases. "Recurrence of *tinea pedis*," Habif et al assure us, "is prevented by wearing wider shoes and expanding the web space with a small strand of lamb's wool (Dr. Scholl's Lamb's Wool)."[54] If a quest for the hypothetical wider shoes seems quixotic, it nonetheless promises to be more focused than the search for the "well-ventilated" or "breathable" shoes that are recommended by most writers. Who makes these things anyway? Thonged sandals which expose the feet to air ought to reduce the odds of dermatophyte incubation, and for people who work at home they may prove practical as well as comfortable. For persons engaged in those high-risk occupations described in Chapter Five (coal miners, telephone linemen, police officers, foot soldiers, et al), open sandal-type footwear on the job is not an option. We may speculate that these workers might be helped somewhat by wearing sandals during their off-duty hours. *Tinea* sufferers, like other people, are probably well-advised to wear "flip-flops" (rubber beach sandals) during visits to swimming pools and communal showers; this measure ought to modestly reduce the likelihood of *T. rubrum* dissemination.

Everybody agrees that persons wearing the customary enclosed shoes or boots should also wear socks or other hosiery, with a view to keeping the feet and the footwear interior as dry as possible. Alas, there is still no consensus regarding the best type of sock or socking for this purpose. The traditional wisdom has called for "cotton or wool socks" which would absorb the moisture inevitably produced by shod feet. But of late some *tinea pedis* gurus have recommended hosiery made of "synthetic fibers" which would supposedly "wick moisture away from the foot." The clinical trial that could resolve this momentous issue has yet to be done. For the time being, absorbent cotton socks continue to look like a more plausible solution than purely synthetic ones. The drawback is that by absorbing moisture from the feet, cotton socks can themselves become extremely damp; they should no doubt be changed if this situation occurs.

Everybody also agrees on the advisability of disinfecting all environmental surfaces and all articles of apparel which might retain *T. rubrum* spores and thus play a role in disease transmission or in reinfection. Like most highly desirable things, this is easier said than done. Bathroom floors, bath tubs, and shower stalls should be cleaned with a potent disinfectant on a regular basis and kept dry when not in use. Ideally, these surfaces would be disinfected every time the barefoot *tinea* sufferer treads upon them, yet this degree of spick-and-span stands to overtax all but the most fanatical housekeepers. The disinfection of a sufferer's socks or stockings seems much more feasible: these items should be washed in warm-to-hot soapy water after each day's use, and then thoroughly dried in the open air or in a rapidly tumbling dryer. That ought to fix *T. rubrum*! A practical strategy for disinfecting a sufferer's shoes would be immensely valuable, because that comfy well-broken-in footwear must be harboring oodles of spores and other viable fungal elements. The most drastic solution has in fact been advocated in print—just throw away all your old shoes and buy new ones! But few physicians would want to propose this expensive exercise to their patients, especially in view of the fact that its effectiveness has not been proven. Several dermatologists at the Veterans Affairs Medical Center in Minneapolis tested a cheaper remedy. They put naphthalene mothballs in the shoes of onychomycosis sufferers and then sealed each pair of shoes "in a plastic bag for four days." No luck! The Red Fungus came out of the mothball bombardment with flying colors, very much alive and ready to reinfect.[55] Athletic *tinea* victims might be advised to put their tennis shoes in a washing machine every so often. The interior of shoes which are not machine-washable can at least be cleaned out periodically with a cloth or paper towel dampened with rubbing alcohol, a sufficiently fungitoxic liquid. After being machine-washed or wiped clean, shoes should be allowed to dry out in the fresh air and sunshine. Will these washing and wiping exercises actually do any good? Heavens, I don't know that—let's just say that these measures can't hurt, are not as messy as the mothballs, and don't require too much of your time and money.

The worm in our disinfection strategies is that they can be only partially successful. Getting *T. rubrum* out of a household is as problematic a task as getting the mosquitoes out of the Florida everglades or the Louisiana bayous. *Fat chance!* But the prospects for sterilizing even a single infected foot are none too good. A standard textbook on microbiology gives us the distressing information that "*T. rubrum* is well suited to survive on the surface of the skin, leading to chronic infection, often for a lifetime."[56] Ouch! No wonder the pharmaceutical companies are doing such a booming business with their "cures" for athlete's foot! The bug just stays on your feet, waiting for the proper incubational conditions to resume its painful inroads. And like the mosquito-control departments down in Dixie, the best you can hope for is not eradication but mitigation. With constant recourse to disinfection procedures and antifungal agents, you might manage to hold the enemy at bay.

The importance of basic hygiene cannot be emphasized enough. If you have mosquitoes in your neighborhood, you don't want to leave buckets of water standing in your backyard: these pests can start breeding in a wet bottle cap. And while we seem to know less about dermatophytes than about mosquitoes, the hygienic measures universally recommended for *tinea* sufferers should never be neglected. Wash your feet at least once daily, being careful to dry the web spaces between your toes. Put on a fresh (clean) pair of socks or stockings whenever you bathe. Since it is not practical to put on a new pair of shoes every day, you should have several pairs and "rotate" them, so that at least you are not wearing the same pair for two days in a row. Give yesterday's sweaty shoes time to dry out, lest they become rapidly overgrown with all manner of fungi.

For years and years I practiced the aforementioned basic hygiene with religious fervor, yet I was never quite free of athlete's foot. Eventually I became aware of a troubling pattern: I would get an outbreak of *tinea pedis* on one foot, and then several weeks later the symptoms would appear *on the other foot*. Something was amiss in these seemingly sensible rituals. After I learned a bit about *T. rubrum* biology, I identified the wolf in sheep's clothing which had probably caused my woes. It was none other than the supposedly friendly **bath towel** used to dry my feet and the web spaces between my toes. *T. rubrum* persists wonderfully well on damp bath towels; of course, that's the reason why jock itch can sometimes spread like wildfire among groups of young male athletes. The guys are not engaging in sexual relations or trading jocks, they're simply passing around a contaminated towel! And the same mode of fungal dissemination implicated in *tinea cruris* (jock itch) also works swimmingly in *tinea pedis* and *tinea unguium*. Under no circumstance should uninfected family members use an unwashed towel recently used by the family's *tinea* sufferer to dry his feet. The cost and bother of providing a separate clean towel for each person will ultimately be far less than that of managing chronic dermatophyte infections for the whole family. Presumably, the risk of disease transmission is greatest when the sufferer has the clinical symptoms of athlete's foot or onychomycosis. We must also presume that a sufferer can inadvertently reinfect himself by using the same bath towel day after day. Hanging a towel on a bathroom hook to dry does not ensure its sterility; even after twenty-four hours it can be the means by which active disease is spread from a symptomatic foot or toe to a seemingly healthy one.

Insofar as towel hygiene is concerned, I have found the most radical solution to be the simplest and the cheapest. I never use a bath towel to dry my feet—I use absorbent paper towels for this purpose, and I take care to use a separate towel for each foot and to dispose of it afterwards. This precaution costs me a few extra pennies each day, yet it should prove less expensive and less troublesome than constantly laundering cloth towels or having to treat frequent outbreaks of athlete's foot. In the long run, however, neither careful foot hygiene nor thorough environmental disinfection, nor both together, is likely to represent an adequate solution to the chronic sufferer's plight.

We should remember that not only has the poor fellow been permanently colonized by the noxious dermatophyte, but that he remains highly susceptible to infection with any new strains of *T. rubrum* he might encounter. The frequent and judicious use of topical antifungals will therefore be as important for *tinea* prevention as the frequent spraying of insecticides has been for mosquito control.

"Can you recommend a good antifungal solution that I might soak my feet in?" I asked my podiatrist friend Doctor S——. "Does somebody make a product which kills the fungus on the skin's surface and stops athlete's foot from recurring so often?" His answer surprised me. "The best thing is white wine vinegar," Doctor S—— said. "Use one tablespoon full for each quart of water; soak your feet for fifteen minutes at a time, twice a day." Long conditioned to the idea that *real* antibiotics had to be pharmaceuticals proven effective in clinical trials and sanctioned by the FDA, I was skeptical. A few hours of surfing the Internet made me more sympathetic to vinegar therapy for athlete's foot: there seemed to be hundreds of websites singing the praises of vinegar, an improbable phenomenon if it had no beneficial effects. Plain old-fashioned vinegar is therefore one folk remedy worthy of serious consideration. Because it is mildly acidic, it can change the skin's pH, creating a surface environment decidedly inhospitable to fungal overgrowths. That vinegar immersions can get *T. rubrum* completely off the feet has not been demonstrated, yet I was becoming extremely interested in any antifungal application which could readily cover an entire foot. Those innovative Miami Beach dermatologists Nardo Zaias and Gerbert Rebell have argued that persons "with distal subungual onychomycosis caused by *T. rubrum*" invariably have a persistent infection on the soles of their feet, even if no symptoms are noticeable there. Thus applying topical antifungals only to the painful lesions in the web spaces, as most sufferers do, probably will not stave off athlete's foot or toenail fungus for any great length of time.[57]

White wine vinegar was starting to smell like a lily. After all, the stuff was cheap, accessible without a prescription, and unlikely to cause side effects other than nauseously reeking tootsies.

But I soon discovered that the world of **alternative medicine** (that's what they're calling folk remedies these days) could be just as aggravating as the standard therapy personified by hyper-busy specialists and super-pricey prescription drugs. The trial data purporting to support the recommended Lamisil and Penlac regimens had been flimsy enough, but there seemed to be no data whatsoever regarding the dose and scheduling of vinegar immersions. What's the optimal proportion of vinegar to water? How often and how long should you soak your feet? Most websites favored higher concentrations than Doctor S— had suggested—say, half vinegar and half water, with the additional hint that the water should be warm for maximal effectiveness and comfort. Straight vinegar dabbed on with a cotton ball was supposed to be the best tonic for those troublesome web-space lesions. Alas, the folksy Internet healers were no more free of commercialism than anybody else. Apple cider vinegar got lauded to the heavens as Mother Nature's special panacea by the very websites offering the stuff for sale. It does taste better than the cheaper white vinegar; that it has superior activity against *T. rubrum* is less certain.

Besides vinegar, there are many other folk remedies for athlete's foot. All manner of herbs, teas, oils, and vitamin supplements have been casually proposed as therapy. And who can say that these things don't work? Dealing with plant-derived "natural" products, alternative-medicine marketers do not need to present data on safety and effectiveness to the FDA. And nobody else has an incentive to do so. The big pharmaceutical companies are not interested in folk remedies, which could never be patented; and few academic pharmacologists would want to stake their careers on the reputed antifungal properties of vinegar, oregano, or garlic. It's all so *infra dig*! The poor *tinea* sufferer should be cautioned that none of these organic substances is likely to have any activity against subungual onychomycosis, where dermatophytes have entrenched themselves under the nail plate. Vinegar soaks—and possibly other folk remedies—can be useful in preventing the recurrence of athlete's foot; the question of cost-effectiveness does not admit of a simple answer. *Per se*, white wine vinegar is cheap; but if you use a quart a day and spend an hour a day soaking your feet in it, your expenditure of time and money will not be inconsequential.

For the vast majority of *tinea* sufferers, the daily use of a **moisture-absorbing antifungal foot powder** should prove to be the cheapest and fastest prophylaxis. Dusting your feet with a powder requires only a few seconds of your time, feels good, and is usually not associated with unpleasant odors or side effects. There are so many foot powders on the market that the author feels impelled to offer a "Consumer Report," drawing upon his considerable personal experience. Back in the early 1990s the antifungal agent in most products was **undecylenic acid**; by the year 2000 many manufacturers had shifted to **miconazole nitrate**, one of the newer drugs of the azole family (this includes clotrimazole, itraconazole, and oxiconazole). Miconazole nitrate is a broad-spectrum agent which can inhibit the growth of other fungal species besides dermatophytes. **Tolnaftate** is a similarly broad-spectrum agent; powder formulations of it have been marketed as **Tinactin®** and under other brand names. All these substances have activity against *T. rubrum* and should be helpful in reducing the frequency of *tinea pedis* outbreaks. Alas, the unbiased clinical trials which would identify the single most effective agent have yet to be done;

individual consumers are therefore free to form their own opinions and to make their own selections. A product's price, availability, tolerability, ease of application, and perceived level of efficacy are factors which every consumer should ponder. The fact that antifungal foot powders are sold over-the-counter does not necessarily mean that long-term daily applications for prophylaxis will be inexpensive. Quite the contrary. I have learned the hard way that some of these products are better buys than others.

Insofar as application is concerned, we may divide the antifungal foot powders into two classes: the **spray powders** which come in metal cans and are applied as a damp aerosol, and the **dry powders** which are shaken out of plastic containers. When they are working as they should, the spray powders can't be beat for convenience. In a second or two you can completely coat those vulnerable web spaces between the toes with a comforting moist powder; this will dry within a minute. Unfortunately, not all manufacturers have the knack for producing a good aerosol powder. I personally want a gentle even spray, and some of these products deliver a sudden blast instead. Oh, the horror stories I could

tell you about defective cans where all the pro-
pellant gas somehow escaped after an application
or two, or where the antifungal liquid leaked out
as large droplets which landed on the floor rather
than on my feet. For years and years I was a big
fan of **Desenex® Spray Powder**; but after the
manufacturer switched from undecylenic acid to
miconazole nitrate, the quality of the spray
seemed to suffer, at least in those cans I tested.
Recently I have been awarding my laurels to
Lotrimin® Spray Powder: although I have
occasionally encountered defective cans, this
product has usually performed well, delivering a
gentle mist of 2% miconazole nitrate at the touch
of a button.

It's easy to get hooked on the convenient
spray powders, but cost-conscious consumers
may be deterred by their price. A modest-sized
can retails for seven dollars or so; and if you
spray your feet twice a day, you'll probably need
a new can after a week or two. Another disadvantage is that the powder coating delivered by
these products is not particularly enduring or
absorbent. If you spray your feet early in the
morning and then examine them at noon, you'll
probably not be able to find the slightest trace

of powder—it's all been washed away! The level of antifungal activity after this happens has unquestionably been reduced and may well be negligible. In terms of price, endurance, and absorbency, the dry powders are by far the best buy. They're much cheaper, and they do a better job of keeping the feet dry. A little container of **Zeasorb®** also retails for seven dollars or so, but then it may last you several months. This dry powder is available in an antifungal formulation (2% miconazole nitrate) as well as a nonmedicated formulation. Both varieties are extremely absorbent and go on working for hours, even on the sweatiest of feet.

The principal disadvantage of dry powders is difficulty of application. The first time I tried to dust the plantar (bottom) surfaces of my feet with Zeasorb, most of the powder landed on the floor. It's so easy to cover those web spaces with a spray powder—simply twist your feet upwards and push the button. But this technique doesn't work with a dry powder, which naturally tends to fall between your toes and keep on going down. One solution is to shake the dry powder into your socks or stockings before pulling them on. That way you'll eventually get most of the powder on your feet. Years ago I often watched my late father shaking foot powder into the tips of his socks; I always wondered why he did that every morning, and now I know. However, my personal technique for Zeasorb application is slightly different. I put the powder on the dorsal surfaces (the tops) of my feet, right where the crevices between the toes begin; and then—just before the powder starts to fall through—I hastily pull on my socks. For safety's sake this maneuver is performed over a wastebasket lined with a plastic bag; after a while that bag reveals quite a powder residue, but at least the stuff isn't on the floor!

Some *tinea pedis* gurus have suggested that you should spray or shake antifungal powder into your shoes. This might help, but it remains far more important to apply the powder directly to your feet. The more areas of the feet dusted, the more effective the prophylaxis stands to be. Therefore unless you are having an unpleasant skin reaction to the powder, you should apply it liberally once or twice a day. Some of the powder trapped within the socks or stockings will filter down into the shoes, serving to combat fungal overgrowths there. Unfortunately, no amount of powdering will give you guaranteed protection against athlete's foot. At best the daily application of an absorbent antifungal powder will reduce the frequency and severity of outbreaks by creating a hostile environment for your resident dermatophytes. That blurb about "curing athlete's foot" which is boldly printed on all the spray powder cans must be taken with a large grain of salt. *Cure my foot! Powders are for prevention!* And they are hardly 100% reliable in this role. I personally subject my feet to a daily powdery pounding as ferocious as the assault on Iwo Jima. First I swoop in low with a can of Lotrimin to hit those fungi-infested web spaces at close range. This is followed by high-altitude aerial bombardment. Holding the Zeasorb above my outstretched toes, I lay down a murderous carpet of white fungicide! Does all this sophisticated weaponry destroy the foe? Not a chance. Every few months *T. rubrum* emerges from its subcutaneous caves to reoccupy the web spaces— and give the lie to those advertising blurbs!

When you do experience the symptoms of resurgent *tinea pedis*, you can rest assured that almost any topical antifungal can produce rapid relief and some measure of control. The key to successful therapy lies largely in the choice of vehicle. Wet formulations (creams, solutions, sprays) are indicated for active disease, because they do a better job of penetrating mycotic skin and killing the deep-burrowing dermatophytes. Powders simply sit on the skin's surface. Insofar as antifungal activity is concerned, topical terbinafine would currently be the agent of choice. The pharmaceutical giant Novartis has been marketing over-the-counter 1% formulations as the **Lamisil AT® Cream**, as the **Lamisil AT® Solution Dropper**, and as the **Lamisil® AT Spray Pump**. While these products may represent the fastest way to get athlete's foot under control, they are not necessarily the most economical. Lured by the spray pump's promise of non-greasy, fast-drying convenience, I put down $12.22 to purchase one at my neighborhood pharmacy. The colorful cardboard box containing this product was certainly spacious—six inches tall and two-and-a-half wide. Alas, the pump itself (contents "1 fl oz") proved to be much smaller than the packaging—I had to root around in the bottom of the box to find it!

The podiatrist Rachel Hart and her colleagues

at the University of Wales have courageously sought to penetrate the haze of exaggerated claims and marketing hoopla that envelopes the topical antifungals used against *tinea pedis*. In an analysis published in the *British Medical Journal*, Hart et al assure us that the costly allylamines (terbinafine belongs to this class) do cure "slightly more fungal infections of the skin of the feet" than other medications. The azole drugs generally took longer (typically four weeks) to achieve control. Yet old-fashioned undecylenic acid proved only slightly less effective than the allylamines and the azoles, and it won the Welsh researchers' laurel for cost-effectiveness. Hart et al concluded that undecylenic acid or one of azoles should be tried first, reserving the allylamines "for treatment failures."[58]

In treating athlete's foot, adequate duration of therapy and adequate expanse of application are as important as the agent used—perhaps even more important. A good recipe for early recurrence is to follow the direction prominently printed on the Lamisil spray-pump box: "one week between the toes." No doubt one week will suffice for symptomatic relief; but if the mycotic skin is thickened and fissured, longer scheduling

would be indicated. Elizabeth S. Martin and Boni
E. Elewski, dermatologists at the University of
Alabama in Birmingham, recommend that the
duration of topical terbinafine therapy for athlete's foot should be "over one week but not over
four weeks." They caution that adjacent asymptomatic areas also need to be treated: "For interdigital *tinea pedis*, patients should apply the topical agent to interdigital areas and soles, because it
is likely that the dermatophyte has infected the
plantar surface. Recurrence is often due to the
patient's discontinuance of medication after
symptoms have abated, but a cure has not occurred."[59]

   Dollar-wise and trouble-wise, the prevention
of recurrent *tinea unguium* is a more pressing
concern than the prevention of recurrent *tinea
pedis*. As we have seen, prolonged *T. rubrum*
infection of the nail bed and matrix can do irreparable damage to the toenails, and its treatment
stands to be far more complicated and expensive
than the treatment of athlete's foot. Once you
have been cured of toenail fungus by investing
thousands in Lamisil and Penlac, how do you

stop that slimy scarlet microbe from gaining re-
entry to the nail unit?   Would that those long-
winded prescribing directives for these two drugs
told us how to prevent future subungual incursions!   But both the pharmaceutical companies
and the academic researchers have been strangely
silent on this point. For shame! While their silence is reproachable, at least it affords the author
an opportunity to offer his own modest suggestions.

Needless to say, newly-cured onychomycosis
patients should begin—and maintain indefinitely
—the previously discussed measures for the control of athlete's foot.   There are additional prophylactic stratagems pertaining specifically to the
toenails which also need to be implemented.
Hygiene is paramount: the toenails should be kept
short, with a view to making them less susceptible to trauma and less hospitable for dermatophytes.   It's best to trim the toenails straight
across, so as to avoid possible irritation of the
lateral grooves and folds. The free edge of the
nail should not project beyond the end of the
digit. Nail enamel (polish) probably should not
be applied to the lady sufferer's toenails, as it
may tend to concentrate moisture beneath the

plates and thus create an environment conducive to fungal growth.

The regular application of a topical antifungal to the toenails and surrounding skin ought to greatly reduce the likelihood of recurrent subungual onychomycosis. Would that one of the pharmaceutical companies made a demonstrably efficacious product for this particular purpose! As it is, nobody seems to have studied this matter properly, and the poor author is left to his own devices. My hunch is that those absorbent dry powders which stave off *tinea pedis* in the web spaces would be much less effective as a prophylaxis against *tinea unguium*. The reason is that subungual onychomycosis typically begins underneath the nail's free edge, in the distal groove where thick keratin-rich skin (the hyponychium) joins with the soft ventral surface of the emerging nail plate. That distal groove is the *Ho Chi Minh Trail* of the Red Fungus! Naturally we would want to saturate this main infiltration route with an agent which has the potential to sink into the hyponychium and which retains its antifungal activity for hours on end. Powder formulations hardly fit this bill: simply getting a dry powder like Zeasorb into the distal grooves would be a dubious enterprise, and we could have little expectation of adherence and penetration. Any wet formulation (cream, lotion, solution, or spray) ought to be a better choice. Over-the-counter **Fungi-Nail®** (25% undecylenic acid in solution), while ineffective against nail bed disease, may have value as a prophylactic treatment for the distal and lateral nail grooves. This product is certainly convenient enough. But Robert Baran of France and his European colleagues have tossed out a different idea: "A weekly application of terbinafine cream in the nail area, between the toes and on the soles of the feet, would be expected to be very effective in preventing reinfection in those individuals who appear to be particularly susceptible to onychomycosis."[60]   Weekly? Twice weekly? Every other day? Daily? Would that somebody would do a clinical trial to establish the optimal agent and the optimal schedule!   In the meantime a cliché must suffice: "Better an ounce of prevention than a pound of cure—*especially with Lamisil.*" If you need a ten-dollar tube of 1% terbinafine cream for a month's prophylaxis, this will nonetheless prove decidedly cheaper than a thirty-day supply of the pricey tablets!!

Eternal Vigilance

must be the cornerstone of any prophylactic strategy. The Red Fungus is posed for perpetual aggression, marching relentlessly throughout the world on billions of feet, yours and mine! We should not expect that this unforgiving foe will be permanently vanquished by any stratagem short of universal amputation, but frequent examination of the toenails in bright sunlight can serve as an early-warning system. At the slightest hint of recurrent discoloration in a nail plate, hie thee to thy dermatologist or podiatrist for a hopefully expert opinion. Suspected fungal incursions on the all-important distal front should be forcefully countered with professional debridement and with what Dr. Baran calls a "transungual delivery system"—viz., a keratophilic antifungal lacquer like Penlac. If accomplished in a timely fashion, will these maneuvers eliminate the need for additional courses of costly oral therapy? Well, we should certainly hope so!

Notes

1. Boni E. Elewski, "Large-scale Epidemiological Study of the Causal Agents of Onychomycosis," *Archives of Dermatology*, 133 (Oct. 1997), pp. 1317-18.

2. "The Dermatophytes" in Elmer W. Koneman et al, *Color Atlas and Textbook of Diagnostic Microbiology*, 5th ed. (Lippincott, 1997), pp. 1019-24.

3. Koneman et al (as in preceding note), p. 1023.

4. *Lifestyle* catalog, Early Spring 2002, p. 32.

5. C. Ralph Daniel III, *Diagnosis of Onychomycosis and Other Nail Disorders: A Pictorial Atlas* (Springer-Verlag New York, 1996), pp. 58-66.

6. Aldo González-Serva, "Structure and Function," in Richard K. Scher and C. Ralph Daniel III, *Nails: Therapy, Diagnosis, Surgery*, 2nd ed. (W. B. Saunders Co., 1997), pp. 12-31.

7. Suthep Jerasutus, "Histology and Histopathology," in Scher and Daniel (as in preceding

note), pp. 55-98.

8. Robert Baran et al, *Onychomycosis: The Current Approach to Diagnosis and Therapy* (London: Martin Dunitz, 1999), pp. 70-71.

9. Boni E. Elewski et al, "Onychomycosis," in Scher and Daniel (as in note 6), pp. 151-62.

10. Baran et al (as in note 8), p. 71.

11. Baran et al (as in note 8), p. 7.

12. Boni E. Elewski et al, "Onychomycosis," in Scher and Daniel (as in note 6), p. 152.

13. David G. Kern, "Occupational Disease," in Scher and Daniel (as in note 6), pp. 282-300.

14. The details of the kaserne's construction are taken from "Wildflecken: A Short History" (U. S. Army Special Services, undated brochure ca. 1970), and "Der Beginn: Truppenübungsplatz und Lager für die deutsche Wehrmacht," accessed at www.rhoenline.de/wta/truppenlager/beginn/htm on July 11, 2002.

15. "Truppenlager und Übungsplatz in Betrieb," accessed at www.rhoenline.de/wta/truppenlager/Betrieb.htm on July 11, 2002.

16. Earl F. Ziemke, *Stalingrad to Berlin: The German Defeat in the East* (Washington: U. S. Army Center of Military History, 1968).

17. Patricia G. Engasser, "Nail Cosmetics,"

in Scher and Daniel (as in note 6), pp. 276-81.

18. Shelley A. Sekula et al, "Nail Salons Can Be Risky Business," *Archives of Dermatology*, 138 (Mar. 2002), pp. 414-15.

19. Engasser (as in note 17), pp. 279-80.

20. Ernst Epstein, "How Often Does Oral Treatment of Toenail Onychomycosis Produce a Disease-Free Nail?" *Archives of Dermatology*, 134 (Dec. 1998), pp. 1551-54.

21. "Lamisil® Tablets: Prescribing Information" (Novartis Pharmaceuticals, April 2001 edition).

22. Roderick J. Hay, *Lamisil: The Evidence* (Parthenon Publishing Group, 2001), p. 80.

23. Michael Hall et al, "Safety of Oral Terbinafine: Results of a Postmarketing Surveillance Study in 25,884 Patients," *Archives of Dermatology*, 133 (Oct. 1997), pp. 1213-19.

24. Discussion of griseofulvin by Boni E. Elewski et al in Scher and Daniel (as in note 6), p. 159.

25. "Pharmacokinetics" in Hay (as in note 22), pp. 12-13.

26. "Prescribing Information" (as in note 21).

27. Kosh Agarwal et al, "Terbinafine and Fulminant Hepatic Failure," *New England Jour-*

nal of Medicine, 340 (Apr. 22, 1999), pp. 1292-93.

28. Trials cited by Hay (as in note 22), p. 77, and in "Prescribing Information" (as in note 21).

29. "Mechanism of Action" in Hay, pp. 9-10, and Novartis data (as in notes 22 and 21).

30. Matthias Bräutigam et al, "Randomised Double-blind Comparison of Terbinafine and Itraconazole for Treatment of Toenail Tinea Infection," *British Medical Journal*, 311 (Oct. 7, 1995), pp. 919-22.

31. "Itraconazole," *Mosby's GenRx*, 10th ed. (Mosby, 2000), Section III, pp. 954-62.

32. "Lamisil® Tablets: Prescribing Information" (April 2001).

33. Piet De Doncker et al, "Antifungal Pulse Therapy for Onychomycosis: Monthly Cycles with Itraconazole," *Archives of Dermatology*, 132 (Jan. 1996), pp. 34-41.

34. E. Glyn V. Evans et al, "Double-blind, Randomised Study of Continuous Terbinafine Compared with Intermittent Itraconazole in Treatment of Toenail Onychomycosis," *British Medical Journal*, 318 (Apr. 17, 1999), pp. 1031-35.

35. Hay (as in note 22), p. 20.

36. Detailed information on ciclopirox nail lacquer has been compiled by Sam Shuster (editor), *Hydroxy-Pyridones as Antifungal Agents with Special Emphasis on Onychomycosis* (Springer-Verlag Berlin, 1999).

37. "Penlac™ Nail Lacquer: Prescribing Information as of August 2000" (package insert), Aventis Pharma Deutschland.

38. *People*, 57 (Jan. 28, 2002), after p. 60.

39. S. Nolting, "Open Studies of Ciclopirox Nail Lacquer in Onychomycosis," in Shuster (as in note 36), pp. 75-80.

40. Richard K. Scher, "Clinical Efficacy of Topical Ciclopirox Nail Lacquer: Double-blind United States Studies on Onychomycosis," in Shuster (as in note 36), pp. 62-68.

41. Penlac package insert (as in note 37).

42. Robert Baran, "Differential Diagnosis of Onychomycosis and Rationale for a Step-Therapy in Treating Nail Fungal Infection," in Shuster (as in note 36), pp. 103-09.

43. Robert Baran, "Topical Amorolfine for 15 Months Combined with 12 Weeks of Oral Terbinafine, a Cost-Effective Treatment for Onychomycosis," *British Journal of Dermatology*, 145 (Oct. 2001), Supplement, pp. 15-19.

44. Penlac package insert (as in note 37).

45. Nolting (as in note 39), pp. 78-79.

46. G. Wozel, "Dose Regimen Studies with Ciclopirox Nail Lacquer," in Shuster (as in note 36), pp. 69-74. Another large German study (1,239 patients) also reported that "after three months of treatment, a once weekly application is sufficient for maintenance therapy." See Nolting (as in note 39), p. 76.

47. Nardo Zaias and Gerbert Rebell, "Onychomycosis Treated Until the Nail Is Replaced by Normal Growth or There Is Failure," *Archives of Dermatology*, 136 (July 2000), p. 940.

48. Isaak Effendy, *Nagelmykosen: Klinik, Diagnose und Therapie* (Thieme Verlag Stuttgart, 2001).

49. Warren S. Joseph, "Podiatric Approach to Onychomycosis," in Scher and Daniel (as in note 6), pp. 301-10.

50. Stuart J. Salasche, "Surgery," in Scher and Daniel (as in note 6), pp. 326-49.

51. Baran et al (as in note 8), p. 49.

52. Philip R. Cohen and Richard K. Scher, "The Nail in Older Individuals," in Scher and Daniel (as in note 6), pp. 127-50. See especially the summaries of "Chemical Modalities for Nail

Avulsion" on pp. 132, 139.

53. "Dermatophyte Infections," *The Merck Manual*, 17th ed. (Merck & Co., 1999), pp. 802-04.

54. Thomas P. Habif et al, "Tinea of the Foot," in *Skin Disease: Diagnosis and Treatment* (Mosby, 2001), pp. 200-03.

55. Erin Warshaw and Debra Ahmed, "Are Mothballs Helpful in Preventing Onychomycosis Reinfection?" *Archives of Dermatology*, 135 (Sept. 1999), pp. 1120-21.

56. Koneman et al (as in note 2), p. 1027.

57. Nardo Zaias and Gerbert Rebell, "Chronic Dermatophytosis Caused by *Trichophyton rubrum*," *Journal of the American Academy of Dermatology*, 35 (Sept. 1996), Supplement, pp. 17-20.

58. Rachel Hart et al, "Systematic Review of Topical Treatments for Fungal Infections of the Skin and Nails of the Feet," *British Medical Journal*, 319 (July 10, 1999), pp. 79-82.

59. Elizabeth S. Martin and Boni E. Elewski, "Tinea Pedis," *eMedicine Journal*, 3 (Jan. 17, 2002), accessed at www.emedicine.com on Aug. 21, 2002.

60. Baran et al (as in note 8), p. 72.

Selective Index of Medical Topics

allylamine drugs, 105, 194
alternative medicine, 183-86
amorolfine nail lacquer, 138-40
artificial nails, 96
athlete's foot (*tinea pedis*): caused by *T. rubrum*,
    12-13; promoted by occlusive footwear, 16-
    17, 65, 92; symptoms, 17-18; medical term
    for, 20; genetic susceptibility to, 61-63;
    communal showers as reservoir, 64-65; high
    incidence among soldiers in South Pacific,
    68; Vietnam fungi-riskier, 69; first docu-
    mented American cases, 173-74; strategies to
    prevent *T. rubrum* infection, 174-99; shoes
    and socks, 175-77; disinfection procedures,
    177-79; *T. rubrum* survives on the skin, 179-
    80; basic hygiene, 180-82; antifungal proper-
    ties of vinegar, 183-86; foot powders, 187-92;
    topical agents evaluated, 192-95; duration of

fingernails (continued):
25, 35; growth rates, 34; function as tools, 41-
42; anatomy of, 43-53; fungal infections of,
92-96
fluorouracil cream, 56-57
folk remedies for athlete's foot, 183-86
foot powders, 187-92
foot soldier: riskiest occupation for *T. rubrum*
onychomycosis, 66-69
free edge of nail, 48-49
Fungi-Nail® (brand name), 24, 28, 123, 198

griseofulvin, 23, 102, 104-05, 165

Habif, Thomas P., 175
Hart, Rachel, 193-94
Hay, Roderick J., 102-04, 106, 117
hepatic function test, 103, 156-57
hyphae: definition of, 18
hyponychium: definition of, 48-49, 197

itraconazole (systemic), 97-99, 104-10, 139, 144-
45. See also Sporanox® capsules.

jock itch (*tinea cruris*), 12-13, 20; spread by bath
 towels, 181
Joseph, Warren S., 166

keratin: protein in skin and nails, 15-16; over-
 production of, 31, 55; absorbs drugs and
 poisons, 44-45; Lamisil and Sporanox highly
 keratophilic, 104-05
keratinocytes, 55
keratoses, 55-56

Lamisil AT® Cream, Solution Dropper, and
 Spray Pump (brand names for topical terbinafine), 193-94, 198
Lamisil® tablets (brand name for terbinafine
 hydrochloride): best systemic antifungal, 25-
 28; Dr. Epstein's estimate of cure rates, 98-
 99; the standard regimens, 100; author experiences sticker shock, 101; side effects, 102-
 04; most effective agent against *T. rubrum*,
 104-07; drug interactions, 108; continuous
 therapy preferred, 109-10; author observes
 drug's action, 110-14; reasons for treatment
 failure, 115-20; author's reservations about